HEALTH WRITER'S HANDBOOK

Barbara Gastel, MD

HEALTH WRITER'S HANDBOOK

Iowa State University Press • Ames

Barbara Gastel, MD, MPH, is associate professor of journalism and medical humanities at Texas A&M University, where she coordinates the master's degree program in science and technology journalism.

∞ Printed on acid-free paper in the United States of America.   First edition, 1998

International Standard Book Number: 0-8138-2113-4

Library of Congress Cataloging-in-Publication Data

Gastel, Barbara.
Health writer's handbook / Barbara Gastel.—1st ed.
p.   cm.
Includes bibliographical references and index.
ISBN 0-8138-2113-4 (alk. paper)
1. Medical writings—Handbooks, manuals, etc.   2. Communication in medicine—Handbooks, manuals, etc.   I. Title.
R119.G376   1998
808'.06661—DC21   97–42038

Last digit is the print number: 9 8 7 6 5 4 3 2 1

CONTENTS

Contents

Contents

Contents

TABLES

ACKNOWLEDGMENTS

Many individuals and institutions contributed directly or indirectly to this book. Gretchen Van Houten of Iowa State University Press encouraged me to pursue my goal of preparing such a work. Texas A&M University granted me leave from my usual duties to do much of the research and writing. Staff of various organizations and government agencies provided material for potential use, and fellow health writers generously shared their experience. Ann A. Duyka, Arkady Mak, Joyce Michel, Jason E. Moore, Carol Cruzan Morton, Anne Woods, and a pair of anonymous reviewers commented helpfully on a draft. Katherine M. Arnold provided valuable help in fact checking. Staff of the Iowa State University Press helped transform the manuscript into the book you see before you.

To all of the above, and to others who aided me in this project, I express my gratitude. I especially thank my husband, Thomas I. Vogel, for his unceasing patience, kindness, and care. To him I dedicate this book.

INTRODUCTION

Many people in many settings now write about health and medicine for general readerships. Yet few have studied medical journalism, and little guidance is readily available in this field.

The current book, which evolved from a course in medical reporting, was written to help address this gap. The book is intended primarily for the beginning or aspiring health writer: the reporter newly assigned to the health beat, the writer newly hired by a medical institution, the clinician hoping to prepare some articles for the public, the student considering a career in the field. More experienced health writers may also encounter new information in this book—as I did while gathering material for it. The book also can assist the occasional health writer: for example, the business writer covering the release of a new drug, the feature writer profiling a clinician or researcher or patient, or the sports writer reporting on an athlete's illness or injury.

Paralleling the writing process, the book begins with guidance in choosing topics, gathering information, and evaluating the information gathered. Next come chapters on crafting the piece. Other areas addressed are presenting information on risk, facing ethical issues, and building a career in health writing. The book also provides basic help in writing about such key realms as heart disease, cancer, infectious disease, and mental health.

Because health writers come from varied backgrounds and have varied goals and tasks, different parts of the book may be of use to different readers. Thus the book has been designed so individual sections can be consulted as needed. Some redundancy has necessarily resulted; it is hoped that those reading the entire book will not find the repetition disruptive.

As readers will notice, this book is oriented largely to the United States and to the print media. Much of the content, however, applies to health writing in other countries. Likewise, much of the book can assist health writers working in the broadcast media and the new electronic media.

Health writing is a vast field—and a rapidly evolving one— especially as

Introduction

computer technologies change the way information is gathered and presented. Thus, suggestions of additions and updates would be very welcome. May we work together to promote health writing of the highest quality.

Barbara Gastel, MD
e-mail: b-gastel@tamu.edu

PART I

Finding Topics and Information

Chapter 1

SOME BASICS

Good health writing begins with choosing a good topic and gathering ample good information. Often the two intertwine: Determining the worth of a topic commonly entails some research, and information gathering often yields ideas for further writing. Thus, this chapter and the four that follow provide guidance in finding both topics and information. The current chapter offers general guidance, including advice on assessing topics and a strategy for gathering information. The remaining four chapters provide help in using specific types of sources, ranging from medical journals to health professionals to the World Wide Web.

Approaches to Finding Topics

The complexity and wonder of the human body. The findings every day in biomedical research. Our changing and challenging health care system. The near-endless array of diseases. Health writers hardly lack subject matter. But how to decide just what to write about?

Depending on their circumstances, health writers vary in the breadth of the decision they face. Freelancers, for example, may be bounded by little more than the ability to match a story to a site. Health writers for the news media also can have considerable scope, though they often must favor material that is newly announced or has a local angle. Health writers working in public information or public relations—say, at a government agency, a medical school, or a disease-related association—typically choose from a narrower range of subjects. Yet they, too, often face considerable choice.

Whatever a health writer's setting, two approaches can work well for finding possible topics. One is to start with questions that people want or need answered. Another is to start by identifying information available to present.

Potential questions to address abound. Listen to the people around you or those in the groups for which you write. What health problems trouble them and their families and friends? What baffles them about their bodies? What concerns them about health care? What questions do they have about keeping healthy? Listen carefully, and also consider what questions you yourself have—or would have in their position. Many topics are likely to suggest themselves.

Likewise, new information on which to base health writing is always becoming available. Thousands of medical journals, some appearing as often as weekly, publish reports of research. Investigators present new findings at medical conferences every day. Expert groups frequently issue health-related recommendations. Drugs and medical devices continually enter the market. New health-care facilities open, and existing ones offer new services. As coming chapters will discuss, information on such developments is readily available.

Evaluating Topics

Indeed, information on what's new in medicine is so readily available that health writers in some settings could keep busy covering nothing else. Publicity materials, such as news releases, deluge health reporters in the popular media, and they are easily obtained by others as well. Over the years, journalists covering science and medicine have repeatedly been criticized for relying so heavily on such materials that they let others set their agendas. Clearly, health writers in media and freelance settings must assess possible topics with care. So must those working in public information and public relations, to ensure that what they present is sound and worthy of attention.

When a potential topic emerges from information you encounter, three basic questions can be useful to consider. First: Is it true? For example, do the researchers' findings solidly support the conclusions? Or, as sometimes occurs, has a news release overstated the findings? Lawrence K. Altman, MD, who writes for *The New York Times*, recalls an instance in which a news release from a major research institute made a preliminary finding seem to be proof of a cure for cancer (Altman 1995).

Second: Is it new? As discussed in chapters to come, written and other sources can aid in determining whether something appearing new is truly so. Such determination can be especially important when a treatment is being hailed as novel. Newness can, however, be in the eye of the beholder. For example, a research finding may have been announced weeks or even months ago in a professional journal. However, if readers of a popular magazine are unaware of the finding, it may be sufficiently fresh.

Third: Is the information important? Often, no absolute answer exists. Rather, the answer may depend on your audience's concerns and your reasons for writing. In popular health writing, as in writing for medical journals (Huth 1990), two useful questions to consider are "So what?" and "Who cares?" If you shrug in response, the topic might best be abandoned.

If your possible topic derives from a question likely to interest your audience, evaluating it includes determining how much of an answer you can provide. Is sufficient information of sufficient quality available to prepare a good piece of writing? If not, do not dismiss the topic entirely. Rather, save it for possible future use. For often the best health writing results when new information emerges to help answer long-important questions.

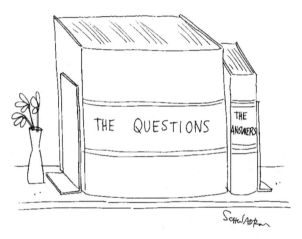

© H.L. Schwadron, reproduced by permission.

Saving Ideas

Often you may come up with a topic that has some merit but is not ready to pursue. A finding may be too preliminary, or adequate information may still be lacking on a question of interest. Or you may be unable to come up with a engaging angle, identify a site for publication, or spend the time the story requires. Do not give up; rather place the idea in an idea file.

You may find it useful to keep two types of idea files: one for mere glimmers of ideas, others for ideas that are more developed. "Glimmer files" contain reminders of various ideas for potential evaluation and pursuit. The reminders may vary in form from a news release you found intriguing, to a journal article on a topic you think bears exploring, to notes from a talk by someone you may wish to profile, to jottings of story ideas that occurred to you after hearing acquaintances discuss medical concerns. Be sure to note in sufficient detail what you have in mind, lest you find yourself wondering after some months, "What is this doing in here?"

Story ideas that are more developed may merit individual files of their own. For example, you may be seriously considering doing a story on a new disease or an increasingly popular type of treatment. As you encounter materials relating to the topic, put them in the file on it.

Later, when you are seeking story ideas, or when new developments may make old topics timely, consult your story files. You may then be off to a running start.

An Information-Gathering Strategy

Once a topic seems promising, information gathering in earnest can begin. Some flexibility still is needed, though: Some topics may not pan out—at least for the present. And sometimes a different focus emerges than initially envisioned.

Good health writing demands thorough research. Not only must such research be deep enough to yield sufficient understanding and ensure that information is solid. Also, it must be broad enough to provide adequate context.

As you do your research, keep careful notes on the sources you use and the information you obtain. Such record-keeping will aid both in writing your piece and in checking it for accuracy.

Following two basic principles can aid in gathering information for health writing efficiently and smoothly. The first is to begin with less technical sources and move to more technical ones. The second is to start with written sources, which may be either printed or electronic, and then move to human sources.

More specifically, basic reference works, such as general and medical dictionaries and encyclopedias, are often good places to start. Next come reading materials for the public. These can include books; magazine, newspaper, and newsletter articles; items on the Internet; and publications of institutions such as government agencies, health-related associations, and companies. In general, the last written sources to consult are books and journals for the medical community.

Finally, interviews with scientists, health professionals, patients, and others can round out the information—and sometimes direct you to additional reading. Also, once you are well prepared, observing surgery or spending time in the laboratory with researchers can garner valuable material for your writing.

The next four chapters, which build on this introduction to finding topics and information, proceed largely in the order outlined here. First comes a chapter on books and periodicals, then one on institutional sources, and finally one on people to interview. Because computerized resources have recently taken a prominent role in gathering information for health writing, they are both noted in these chapters and discussed in a separate chapter.

Chapter 2

BOOKS AND PERIODICALS

Good health writers are good health readers. Knowledgeable about medical books and journals, they draw on such resources to generate story ideas, assess those ideas, and gather information for their writing. This chapter provides guidance in approaching the medical literature. Given the growing availability of computerized resources in libraries and elsewhere, it touches on materials in electronic formats as well as those in print.

General and Medical Libraries

General and medical libraries offer health writers a wealth of information and guidance. Knowing and using these libraries well is a mark of the truly professional health writer.

Given the importance of medical subjects to the population, public libraries often have good collections on health. Especially when you are approaching a new topic, such libraries can be a fine place to start. Consider beginning in the reference section. Reference sources, such as general encyclopedias and the *McGraw-Hill Encyclopedia of Science and Technology* (1997), often provide a good grounding; you can then move to medical encyclopedias and other more specialized reference works.

Popular books and articles available at public libraries can introduce your topic in more detail or provide more up-to-date information. If an area is new to you, consider beginning with books written for young adults; then move to other books and to popular articles, which you can identify through the *Readers' Guide to Periodical Literature* or computerized literature-search systems. You may also be able to consult materials such as publications from the National Institutes of Health, especially if the library has a government documents section. In larger libraries, you can look at materials that are more technical, such as basic medical textbooks and major medical journals. If a public library lacks materials you are seeking, it may be able to borrow them from another library through interlibrary loan. As well as providing printed items, the library may offer use of

I. Finding Topics and Information

computerized information sources to which you would not otherwise have access.

The main libraries of nearby colleges and universities also are likely to have collections that can aid you. If you are not enrolled or employed at the college or university, you may not be able to borrow books. However, you may still be able to consult and photocopy materials from the library.

To explore the medical literature in some depth, a medical library generally is a must. Not only will you have access to many medical books and journals, you will also have indexes needed to find articles on your topic. And importantly, you will have medical librarians who can aid you in your search.

Fortunately, the United States has an extensive system of medical libraries. Typically, the most suitable medical library for a health writer is that at a nearby medical school. If you are not near a medical school, or if you are uncertain which medical library is most suitable, you can call the National Network of Libraries of Medicine at 1-800-338-7657. Also, Volume 2 of the *Medical and Health Information Directory* (Boyden 1994) lists medical libraries in the United States and Canada.

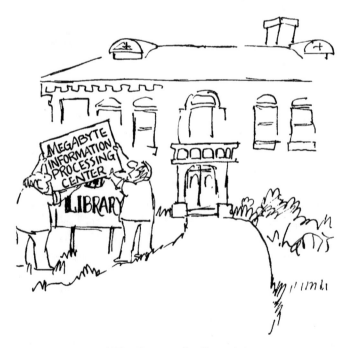

© Sidney Harris, reproduced by permission.

2. Books and Periodicals

To make the most of general and medical libraries, invest the time in getting to know them well. If tours are available, take them; perhaps take them twice. Ditto for demonstrations that libraries offer on searching the literature.

Also, get to know the librarians at your medical library. When you have questions, ask. And let the librarians know what you are working on. Given their familiarity with the literature, they may often direct you to resources you did not know to seek. "They'll go out of their way to help you find what you need," an experienced health writer observes. "Ultimately, your success is theirs, too." (Scully and Scully 1986, 90)

Medical libraries, and medical collections at general libraries, often are busy, which can frustrate the health writer trying to gather information for a story. At peak times you may well have to wait for access to a computer terminal or photocopying machine. To help avoid such frustration, check what times tend to be least busy. You may find, for instance, that a medical school library is relatively empty in the early morning, when most of the students and physicians are in class or visiting hospital patients.

Although libraries aid mainly in gathering information for stories, they also can be sources of story ideas. At general and medical libraries, look at displays of new books; some may suggest story ideas to you. At medical libraries, also browse through journals on the current periodicals rack. And when doing research for writing projects, be alert for material that may generate spinoff stories.

As you keep using libraries for your health writing, you may find sources that you use repeatedly. Consider obtaining these items for your personal library. Many basic medical books are available at general bookstores. Others can be obtained at medical bookstores, which often are located at or near medical schools. Such books also can be readily ordered from publishers. Medical journals and newsletters generally contain information on subscribing. If in doubt, once again, consult your librarian.

Medical Books

Key Reference Books

Many excellent medical reference books are available for health writers to consult. Among the most basic are medical dictionaries. The giants in the field, both literally and figuratively, are *Dorland's Illustrated Medical Dictionary* (1994) and *Stedman's Medical Dictionary* (1995), each of which appears in a new edition every several years. Pocket editions are available of both of these medical dictionaries, and other less extensive but helpful dictionaries are published as well. In addition to being available at libraries, various medical dictionaries are widely sold at bookstores. For the serious health writer they can be a fine investment.

Home or family medical encyclopedias, such as the *American Medical Association Family Medical Guide* (Clayman 1994), also can serve the health writer well. A standard, more technical compendium is *The Merck Manual* (Berkow 1992), first published in 1899. Although geared to physicians, this chunky work covering disorders of every body system makes a fine desk reference for the health writer. An online version can be accessed on the World Wide Web at http://www.merck.com.

For information on pharmaceuticals, a key reference work is the *Physicians' Desk Reference* (1997), commonly known as the *PDR*. Published annually, the *PDR* provides information on prescription drugs available in the United States. Additional information on prescription and nonprescription drugs may be obtained from various other readily available reference works.

Good reference works also exist in other, more specialized areas of medicine and health. Some such books, or types thereof, are noted in the following section. Selected others are mentioned in Chapter 10, which deals with covering some specific areas of health.

If you are seeking reference works, sources of further direction include the book *Introduction to Reference Sources in the Health Sciences* (Roper and Boorkman 1994), published by the Medical Library Association. Also, the *Harvard Health Letter,* a newsletter for the public, has published articles (Thomas 1993, Gillyatt 1996) recommending medical reference books and other information-gathering resources.

Other Helpful Medical Books

Textbooks in various medical specialties—such as internal medicine, pediatrics, and surgery—offer more detailed overviews of medical conditions and their treatment than do reference works listed above. The best and most up-to-date such books generally are available in reference sections of medical libraries. Elsewhere in medical libraries you can find *monographs*—that is, books dealing in depth with individual diseases or other specialized medical subjects.

2. Books and Periodicals

Good health writing often looks beyond the purely biomedical, putting its subject in broader context. Check reference and other sections of libraries for works containing material on historical, social, economic, ethical, and other aspects of medicine. Examples of such works include *The Cambridge World History of Human Disease* (Kiple 1993) and the *Encyclopedia of Bioethics* (Reich 1995).

Also, you may be seeking ideas for illustrating your work. Illustrations in medical books can yield ideas. In addition, the works can be sources of illustrations themselves. To reprint illustrations, typically permission must be obtained from the publisher or other copyright holder; sometimes a fee must be paid. However, some sources, such as U.S. government publications and *The Sourcebook of Medical Illustration* (Cull 1989), do not bear such restrictions. Keeping alert for illustration ideas early in an information search and placing the ideas in a file can save effort later.

Strengths and Limitations of Medical Books

Medical books are good for some things but not for others. Given their scope, they function well in providing overviews of subjects. Many contain bibliographies or reference lists useful in seeking further information. And looking at medical books can aid in identifying experts to interview: Because authors of medical books and chapters have broad and authoritative grasps of their subjects and generally know many people in their fields, they can be good to interview and to contact for suggestions of others to consult.

The main limitation of medical books is that, given the publication process, they cannot include the most recent information. Although books in computerized format may be more up-to-date than their printed counterparts, they are rarely as current as periodicals. Nor do they typically deal in depth with specific pieces of research. Thus, the health writer's information search generally must proceed to periodicals, the subject of the rest of this chapter.

Medical Periodicals

Some Taxonomies of Medical Periodicals

Medical periodicals are a rather diverse lot. Knowing some of the differences can aid in seeking topics and information. One distinction is be-

I. Finding Topics and Information

tween general and specialized medical journals. Another is between journals containing reports of new research and those devoted to summarizing what is already known. And a third is between medical journals and other periodicals, such as newsletters, for the medical profession.

Two major general medical journals are published in the United States. One is *JAMA:* the *Journal of the American Medical Association,* issued 48 times a year. The other is the *New England Journal of Medicine,* which appears every week. Both journals feature original reports of research and contain other types of articles as well. Some material from each journal is available on the World Wide Web, at http://www.ama-assn.org and http://www.nejm.org, respectively. The major general medical journals in Britain are the *BMJ (British Medical Journal)* and *The Lancet*; in Canada it is the *Canadian Medical Association Journal.*

As almost anyone reading U.S. newspapers or tuning in to the U.S. broadcast media may discern, *JAMA* and the *New England Journal of Medicine* are major sources of medical news in the United States. Some (for example, Houn et al. 1995) have criticized journalists' extensive, and sometimes nearly exclusive, reliance on these two sources. The considerable coverage of research in these journals, however, does have some justification. As general medical journals, *JAMA* and the *New England Journal* strive to publish material of broad appeal to the medical profession; thus, they are more likely to contain findings of public interest than, say, a journal of ophthalmology or urology. Both journals also are known for their high standards. Because both journals appear so frequently, much material from them is available. And both journals facilitate coverage by health writers; early copies of each are available to journalists, and *JAMA* also provides news releases on some articles.

As a health writer, you can hardly neglect *JAMA* and the *New England Journal* in your search for story ideas. However, you do well to venture further, to more specialized and less frequently published journals. Unless you work in the daily or weekly media, you probably need not scurry to find articles in specialty journals as soon as they come out. Rather you can periodically scan journals in various specialties. Besides seeking story ideas in medical specialty journals (for example, in pediatrics or surgery), look at journals in areas such as public health, medical education, hospital administration, and health policy. Some examples of prominent journals are listed in Table 2-1.

In addition to medical journals, general scientific journals can be worth scanning. One such journal is *Science,* published weekly by the

Table 2-1:   Some Prominent Medical Journals

Listed below are the journals indexed in the *Abridged Index Medicus*, which contains citations from about 120 journals of particular interest to practicing physicians. These leading journals tend to be good sources for health writers to use as well.

Academic Medicine
AJR: American Journal of Roentgenology
American Family Physician
American Heart Journal
American Journal of Cardiology
American Journal of Clinical Nutrition
American Journal of Clinical Pathology
American Journal of the Medical Sciences
American Journal of Medicine
American Journal of Nursing
American Journal of Obstetrics and Gynecology
American Journal of Ophthalmology
American Journal of Pathology
American Journal of Physical Medicine and Rehabilitation
American Journal of Psychiatry
American Journal of Public Health
American Journal of Respiratory and Critical Care Medicine
American Journal of Surgery
American Journal of Tropical Medicine and Hygiene
Anaesthesia
Anesthesia and Analgesia
Anesthesiology
Annals of Emergency Medicine
Annals of Internal Medicine
Annals of Otology, Rhinology and Laryngology
Annals of Surgery
Annals of Thoracic Surgery
Archives of Dermatology
Archives of Disease in Childhood
Archives of Disease in Childhood, Fetal and Neonatal Edition

Archives of Environmental Health
Archives of General Psychiatry
Archives of Internal Medicine
Archives of Neurology
Archives of Ophthalmology
Archives of Otolaryngology—Head and Neck Surgery
Archives of Pathology and Laboratory Medicine
Archives of Pediatrics and Adolescent Medicine
Archives of Physical Medicine and Rehabilitation
Archives of Surgery
Arthritis and Rheumatism

Blood
BMJ [British Medical Journal]
Brain
British Heart Journal
British Journal of Obstetrics and Gynaecology
British Journal of Radiology
British Journal of Rheumatology
British Journal of Surgery

Ca: A Cancer Journal for Clinicians
Canadian Medical Association Journal
Cancer
Chest
Circulation
Clinical Orthopaedics and Related Research
Clinical Pediatrics
Clinical Pharmacology and Therapeutics
Critical Care Medicine
Current Problems in Surgery

Diabetes
Digestive Diseases and Sciences

Table 2-1: *(continued)*

Disease-a-Month

Endocrinology

Gastroenterology
Geriatrics
Gut

Heart and Lung
Hospital Practice
Hospitals and Health Networks

JAMA [Journal of the American Medical Association]
Journal of Allergy and Clinical Immunology
Journal of the American College of Cardiology
Journal of the American College of Surgeons
Journal of the American Dietetic Association
Journal of Bone and Joint Surgery, American Volume
Journal of Bone and Joint Surgery, British Volume
Journal of Clinical Endocrinology and Metabolism
Journal of Clinical Investigation
Journal of Clinical Pathology
Journal of Family Practice
Journal of Gerontology
Journal of Immunology
Journal of Infectious Diseases
Journal of Laboratory and Clinical Medicine
Journal of Laryngology and Otology
Journal of Nervous and Mental Disease
Journal of Neurosurgery
Journal of Nursing Administration
Journal of Oral and Maxillofacial Surgery
Journal of Pediatrics
Journal of Thoracic and Cardiovascular Surgery

Journal of Toxicology: Clinical Toxicology
Journal of Trauma
Journal of Trauma, Injury, Infection, and Critical Care
Journal of Urology
Journals of Gerontology. Series A, Biological Sciences and Medical Sciences
Journals of Gerontology. Series B, Psychological Sciences and Social Sciences

Lancet

Mayo Clinic Proceedings
Medical Clinics of North America
Medical Letter on Drugs and Therapeutics
Medicine

Neurology
New England Journal of Medicine
Nursing Clinics of North America
Nursing Outlook
Nursing Research

Obstetrics and Gynecology
Orthopedic Clinics of North America

Pediatric Clinics of North America
Pediatrics
Physical Therapy
Plastic and Reconstructive Surgery
Postgraduate Medicine
Progress in Cardiovascular Diseases
Public Health Reports

Radiologic Clinics of North America
Radiology

Southern Medical Journal
Surgery
Surgical Clinics of North America

Urologic Clinics of North America

Western Journal of Medicine

SOURCE: *Abridged Index Medicus*. Volume 26. 1995. Bethesda, MD: National Library of Medicine.

2. Books and Periodicals

American Association for the Advancement of Science. As well as containing reports of biomedical and other research, *Science* has a news section helpful in following research trends and policy issues. Another general scientific journal drawn on by health writers is the British journal *Nature*.

Increasingly, medical and scientific journals are presenting material online as well as on paper (Taubes 1996a). Some offer news releases or other supplementary matter online or offer links to related articles. Some new journals are appearing exclusively in online form.

Various resources can aid in seeking recently published journal articles that can spark ideas for stories. One is *Current Contents,* a weekly collection of journals' tables of contents; long available in print, it also is now available online. Another helpful publication is *Science News: The Weekly Newsmagazine of Science,* which often includes articles on studies newly reported in medical journals. Also useful to consult are the abstracts (summaries) that *JAMA* publishes of articles that have appeared in other journals in the United States and abroad. Newsletters offering health professionals summaries of articles recently appearing in various journals can aid the health writer as well. One such periodical is *Journal Watch,* which includes highlights from various major journals. More specialized newsletters, such as *Journal Watch for Psychiatry* and the American Psychological Association publication *Clinician's Research Digest,* also can prove helpful.

Not all medical journals contain reports of new research; some focus instead on giving clinicians practical overviews. Some people look down on such nonresearch journals. And some such journals truly are little more than carriers for advertisements. However, the better journals—for example, *Hospital Practice* and *American Family Physician*—can be fine resources. Health writers can fruitfully draw on them to obtain background information, identify trends or developments on which to write, and find experts to interview.

Medical periodicals other than journals also can be good resources for health writers. One such periodical is the *Morbidity and Mortality Weekly Report,* published by the federal Centers for Disease Control and Prevention. The *MMWR,* which contains reports of outbreaks and other material on public health, is available in print and on the World Wide Web (via http://www.cdc.gov/; Adobe Acrobat reader required). Selected items from the *MMWR* also are reprinted in *JAMA.* Another well regarded periodical is *The Medical Letter on Drugs and Therapeutics,* a newsletter providing reports on pharmaceuticals. Both publications can be good sources of background information and story ideas.

I.   Finding Topics and Information

Anatomy of a Medical Journal

Medical journals vary somewhat in anatomy. However, some commonalities exist among journals containing reports of new research. Knowing these commonalities can aid in using medical journals to identify possible topics and gather information.

The reports of new research—sometimes bearing such labels as "Original Articles" or "Original Contributions"—typically form the core of journals containing such reports. (See Figure 2-2 for a sample table of contents from *JAMA*.) With rare exceptions, each such report is written in the "IMRAD format": Introduction, Methods, Results, and Discussion. The introduction provides background and identifies the question the research addressed. The methods section then describes how the research was conducted. The results section presents the findings; often it contains tables or illustrations. And the discussion interprets the findings; among items that may be discussed are the relationship of the current findings to those of other researchers, the limitations of the research, and the implications of the findings for clinical practice or public health. Typically, each article is preceded by an abstract summarizing it. References to other writings appear at the end of the article.

This standard format lets readers—including health writers—know where to seek what type of information. If an article seems promising from the title and abstract, some health writers scan the article from beginning to end to see whether it is of sufficient interest to merit more careful inspection. Others begin by looking at the introduction and discussion; if these sections suggest that the article has sufficient appeal, the methods and results sections are then reviewed to provide some indication of the strength of the research. As will be discussed in Chapter 6, articles still seeming suitable to write about should then undergo more thorough and critical review.

Often, the most appealing articles to write about are those that report striking findings. Journalists tend (see, for instance, Koren and Klein 1991) to neglect other articles—for example, those showing that a treatment is ineffective or suggesting that an agent poses little or no risk. The dilemma is a difficult one. If three studies arrive at results favoring a treatment and another three indicate that the treatment has no effect, writing articles only about the former will give a distorted impression. Yet in general, articles saying that something makes little difference are not deemed very newsworthy. One solution can be to prepare an article discussing all six

Figure 2-2: **Table of Contents from the *Journal of the American Medical Association***

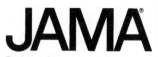

The Journal of the American Medical Association
113 Years of Continuous Publication
World Wide Web Address: http://www.ama-assn.org
EDITORIAL STAFF
Editor: George D. Lundberg, MD
Deputy Editor: Richard M. Glass, MD
Deputy Editor (West): Drummond Rennie, MD
Senior Editors: Phil B. Fontanarosa, MD, Margaret A. Winker, MD
Senior Contributing Editor: M. Therese Southgate, MD
Contributing Editors: Charles B. Clayman, MD, Helene M. Cole, MD, Thomas B. Cole, MD, MPH, David S. Cooper, MD, Harriet S. Meyer, MD, Carin M. Olson, MD, Jeanette M. Smith, MD, Jody W. Zylke, MD
Consulting Editors: Roger C. Bone, MD, Robert A. Clark, MD
Statistical Editor: Naomi Vaisrub, PhD
Associate Senior Editor: Annette Flanagin
Associate Editors: Charlene Breedlove, Roxanne K. Young
Fishbein Fellow: David H. Mark, MD, MPH
Medical News and Humanities: Phil Gunby (director)
Medical News & Perspectives: Marsha F. Goldsmith (editor); Charles Marwick, Andrew Skolnick, Joan Stephenson, PhD, Rebecca Voelker (associate editors)
Assistant Editors: Brian P. Pace, Kate Whetzle
EDITORIAL BOARD
Daniel M. Albert, MD, Madison, Wis
Kenneth A. Arndt, MD, Boston, Mass
H. David Banta, MD, Amsterdam, the Netherlands
Jack D. Barchas, MD, New York, NY
Robert J. Blendon, ScD, Boston, Mass
Marjorie A. Bowman, MD, MPA, Winston-Salem, NC
James E. Dalen, MD, Tucson, Ariz
Catherine D. DeAngelis, MD, Baltimore, Md
Lois DeBakey, PhD, Houston, Tex
R. Gordon Douglas, Jr, MD, New York, NY
Ronald G. Evens, MD, St Louis, Mo
William H. Foege, MD, Atlanta, Ga
Michael E. Johns, MD, Baltimore, Md
Colin I. Johnston, MB,BS, Melbourne, Australia
Robert J. Joynt, MD, PhD, Rochester, NY
Max Just, MD, Basel, Switzerland
Donald A. B. Lindberg, MD, Bethesda, Md
William W. McLendon, MD, Chapel Hill, NC
Arno G. Motulsky, MD, Seattle, Wash
Quan Dong Nguyen, MD, Boston, Mass
Claude H. Organ, Jr, MD, Oakland, Calif
Michael Peckham, MB, MD, London, England
Edmund D. Pellegrino, MD, Washington, DC
Uwe E. Reinhardt, PhD, Princeton, NJ
Povl Riis, MD, Copenhagen, Denmark
Wolf-J. Stelter, MD, Frankfurt, Germany
Masaaki Terada, MD, Tokyo, Japan
INTERNATIONAL ADVISORY COMMITTEE
Bassel Atallah, MD, JAMA—Middle East
Demetre I. Athanassiadis, MD, JAMA—Greece
Mauro Bologna, MD, JAMA—Italy
Miguel Vigeant Gomes, MD, JAMA—Portugal
Yuichiro Goto, MD, JAMA—Japan
Ragini Jain, MD, JAMA—India
Evin Kantemir, MD, JAMA—Turkey
A. J. Khan, SI, FRCP, JAMA—Pakistan
Jin-Pok Kim, MD, JAMA—Korea
C. R. Kumana, MBBS, JAMA—Southeast Asia
Li Chengyi, MD, JAMA—China
Maria S. P. da Silva, MD, JAMA—Brazil
Miguel Vilardell Tarres, MD, JAMA—Spanish Language
Ivan Vidmar, MD, JAMA—Slovenia
Jiří Widimský, MD, DrSc, JAMA—Czech/Slovak

JAMA (ISSN 0098-7484) is published weekly by the American Medical Association, except for 4 combined issues in months with 5 Wednesdays. Address: 515 N State St, Chicago, IL 60610.
SUBSCRIPTION RATES—The subscription rate for AMA members ($20 per year) is included in and is not deductible from the annual AMA membership dues. The annual subscription rates for nonmembers are $125 in the United States and US possessions, $160 in the Americas, and £110 outside the Americas. The rate for nonmember medical students and resident physicians is $80 in the United States. The annual institution rates are $160 in the United States, $200 in the Americas, and £145 outside the Americas. Address all subscription communications to: Subscriber Services Center, American Medical Association, PO Box 10946, Chicago, IL 60610. Phone: (800) 262-2350; Fax: (312) 464-5831; e-mail: ama-subs@web.ama-assn.org.
CHANGE OF ADDRESS—POSTMASTER, send all address changes to: JAMA, The Journal of the American Medical Association, attention: Subscription Department, PO Box 10946, Chicago, IL 60610. Notification of address change must be made at least 6 weeks in advance; include both old and new addresses and a recent mailing label. Periodicals postage paid at Chicago and at additional mailing offices. GST Registration Number: 12622 5556 RT.
JAMA® Registered in the US Patent and Trademark Office.
Copyright© 1996 by the American Medical Association

December 18, 1996, Vol 276, No. 23   Pages 1853-1924
To promote the science and art of medicine and the betterment of the public health.

Original Contributions

Special Communication

Brief Report

Review

Editorials

(Table of Contents continued on next page.)

19

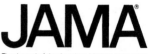

JAMA

The Journal of the American Medical Association

SCIENTIFIC INFORMATION AND MULTIMEDIA STAFF

New Media: William M. Silberg (editorial director), Marty Suter (assistant editor)
Editorial Systems and Administration: Elaine Williams (director), Vee Bailey (electronic input specialist)
Administrative Assistant: Helga Fritz
Editorial Assistants: Patricia Joworski, Gale Saulsberry, Juliana Walker (group supervisors); Kemberly Evans (letters coordinator); Linda Baker, Mary Cannon, Lenette Gardner, Shirley Gogins, Gwenn Gregg, Lisa Hardin, Sharon Iverson, Mary Ann Lilly, Ethel Pinkston, Raul Serrato, Gloria Tate
Editorial Processing Division: Cheryl Iverson (director), Diane L. Cannon (freelance manager), Pete Johlie (assistant freelance coordinator). Paul Frank (senior copy editor/Atex specialist)
Copy Editors: Jane C. Lantz (director), Susan R. Benner (senior copy editor), Fiona M. Bruce, Bill Clements, Susan Goeks

PRODUCTION AND DISTRIBUTION STAFF

Production and Distribution Division: Mary C. Steermann (director), Bonnie Van Cleven (manager, budgets and costs), Vanessa Hayden (director, advertising and production), Linda Knott (director, electronic production), Mary Ellen Johnston (electronic coordinator), Melanie Parenti (database assistant)
Managers: Susan Price (print production), Teresa Omiotek (proofreading), Carole Piszker (advertising), Charl Richey-Davis (color and graphics), Sandra Lopez (composition & pagination)
Proofreaders: David Antos, Daniel James, Mary Kay Tinerrila
Production Associates and Operators: Karen Adams-Taylor, Gail Barrett, Karen Branham, Debbie Camp, Brenda Chandler-Haynes, Michael L. Culbert, Betty Frigerio, Mary Ann Kuranda, Sarah Powell, Jeni Reiling, Christine M. Wagenknecht, JoAnne Weiskopf, Alicja Wojcik
Production Assistants: Ruth Sprague, Jo Anne Turner

CIRCULATION AND MARKETING STAFF

Circulation Processing: Beverly Martin (director)
Circulation Development: Ann Westerbeke (director)
Licensing and Permissions: Norman Frankel (director), Kathy Gaydar (indexing), Ada Jiminez-Walker (permissions)
Reprint Coordinator: Joseph Rekash

AMA Officers

President: Daniel H. Johnson, Jr, MD*
President-Elect: Percy Wootton, MD*
Immediate Past President: Lonnie R. Bristow, MD
Secretary-Treasurer: Randolph D. Smoak, Jr, MD*
Speaker, House of Delegates: Richard F. Corlin, MD
Vice-Speaker, House of Delegates: John A. Knote, MD

AMA Trustees

Regina M. Benjamin, MD (Young Physician); Yank D. Coble, Jr, MD; Nancy W. Dickey, MD* (Chair); Timothy T. Flaherty, MD*; Palma E. Formica, MD; Michael S. Goldrich, MD (Resident); J. Edward Hill, MD; William E. Jacott, MD; D. Ted Lewers, MD*; William H. Mahood, MD; John C. Nelson, MD; Donald J. Palmisano, MD, JD; Pamela Petersen-Crair (Student); Thomas R. Reardon, MD* (Vice-Chair); Randolph D. Smoak, Jr, MD*
*Executive Committee.

AMA EXECUTIVE STAFF

Executive Vice President: P. John Seward, MD
Deputy Executive Vice President: Kenneth E. Monroe
Group Vice President, Business and Management Services: James F. Rappel
Editor in Chief, Scientific Information and Multimedia: George D. Lundberg, MD
Vice President, Publishing: Peter J. Murphy
Publisher: Robert L. Kennett
Publisher, New Media: Michael D. Springer

ADVERTISING OFFICES—Eastern: 119 Cherry Hill Road, 3rd Floor, Parsippany, NJ 07054 (Representatives: Alice H. Herman, Stuart H. Williams [201-263-9191]); **Midwest/Farwest:** 515 N State St, Chicago, IL 60610 (Representative: Jeffery J. Bonistalli [312-464-2551]); **Physician Recruitment Advertising:** 312-464-2456

ADVERTISING PRINCIPLES—Advertisements in this issue have been reviewed to comply with the principles governing advertising in AMA publications. A copy of these principles is available on request. The appearance of advertising in AMA publications is not an AMA guarantee or endorsement of the product or the claims made for the product by the manufacturer.

MANUSCRIPT SUBMISSION—Send manuscripts to the Editor, George D. Lundberg, MD, JAMA, 515 N State St, Chicago, IL 60610.

All articles published, including editorials, letters, and book reviews, represent the opinions of the authors and do not reflect the official policy of the American Medical Association or the institution with which the author is affiliated, unless this is clearly specified.

Reprinted with permission.

2 0

studies and considering why the results may have differed. Another can be to present each new positive study in the context of all the studies that have gone before. Once again, providing context is a mark of good health writing.

In some journals, editorials by experts provide broader perspective on the research reported. In seeking context for a research article, see whether an editorial about it appears in the same issue of the journal. And in seeking story ideas, also look at other editorials in the journal, as well as the "sounding boards" or other opinion pieces that the journals publish.

Many journals contain *review articles*—that is, articles summarizing what is known about a given topic. Traditionally, these articles have resembled book chapters reviewing the literature. More recently some such articles, known as *metaanalyses,* have combined quantitative data from various studies in search of more definitive conclusions. Review articles are popular with physicians, who find them an efficient way to stay up to date. Similarly, for health writers, review articles can be excellent sources of background and context. Some review articles—for example, those on new procedures or recent trends—also can be sources of story ideas.

A glance at the book review section of a journal, and at the books-received listing, also can yield story ideas. The topics of the books can suggest topics for future stories. In general medical journals, especially, some of the books are for general readerships and thus are well suited to review for popular media. The book review section can call attention to books useful as sources of background. Also, the review sections of some journals evaluate computerized resources, which can interest or assist the health writer.

Letters to the editor also can be worth a look. They can aid in following controversies in medicine. Sometimes the letters report amusing ailments—such as Frisbee finger, jogger's nipples, and waterskier's enema (Moskow 1987)—that can be the subject of humorous stories for the popular media.

Some journals, such as *JAMA,* also contain news sections, which can yield story ideas. In addition, conference announcements in journals can provide leads to pursue. And for the astute health writer, even the classified advertisements can suggest areas to explore.

Physiology of Peer-Reviewed Journals

To work with journals, it is helpful to know how journals work. In particular, it's helpful to know how reports of new research are chosen for pub-

I. Finding Topics and Information

lication. Central to this selection mechanism is a process known as *peer review*. When investigators submit a manuscript on their research for potential publication in a journal, the editor of the journal typically sends copies of the manuscript to two or more experts in the research area—in other words, "peers" of the authors. These peer reviewers are instructed to evaluate the manuscript's suitability for publication and to report to the editor on the strengths and weaknesses they perceive. Based on the peer reviewers' feedback and the editor's own assessment of the manuscript, the editor reaches a decision. Sometimes the decision is not to publish the article (in which case the authors can submit the manuscript to another journal for potential publication). Rarely is a manuscript accepted for publication as is. More often, the authors are asked to make various revisions and then resubmit the manuscript.

For the health writer, this evaluation process has various implications. Peer review and editorial review help ensure that only sound research is published; thus, checking whether a given piece of research has been reported in a peer-reviewed journal can aid in deciding whether to write about it. (It should be noted, though, that peer-reviewed journals vary in their standards. Also, because a study often reveals only a small part of the big picture, research can be well done but yield conclusions that later prove untrue.) In addition, the review and subsequent revision that manuscripts undergo often result in better, more informative articles in journals—and thus articles that are more useful to the health writer.

However, the time needed for the evaluation process—and beforehand for writing the article, and afterward for editing and publishing it—often means that many months elapse between the time research is completed and the time it is reported in a journal. One question that arises is whether health writers should release stories on the research during this lag time. As noted below, different sources have different answers.

Pre-publication Publicity: Embargoes, etc.

Some journals place embargoes on the articles they publish. In other words, they prohibit the media from releasing stories about the articles until the official publication date of the issue in which the articles appear (or until late the previous day). Publishers of journals with embargoes state that the embargoes allow physicians time to read about research before it is widely publicized. Some advocates also note that the embargoes give journalists sufficient time to prepare their stories carefully, rather

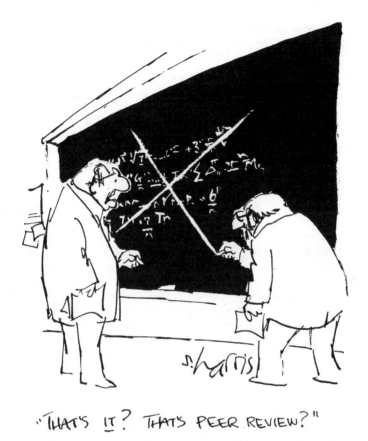

"THAT'S IT? THAT'S PEER REVIEW?"

than racing to see who can break the story first. It also has been contended, however, that journals place embargoes in part to maintain their own newsworthiness.

The International Committee of Medical Journal Editors, consisting mainly of editors of leading medical journals, has issued a statement on medical journals and the popular media (1993). This statement, shown in Figure 2-4, calls for authors not to publicize their work before it appears in a journal. However, it notes that special arrangements can be made when earlier dissemination of the information is important to public health. This statement does not discourage reporters from writing about unpublished research presented at conferences, but it does discourage researchers from giving reporters more detailed information than included

Figure 2-4: Medical Journals and the Popular Media (Statement from the International Committee of Medical Journal Editors)

The public's interest in news of medical research has led the popular media to compete vigorously to get information about research as soon as possible. Researchers and institutions sometimes encourage the reporting of research in the popular media before full publication in a scientific journal by holding a press conference or giving interviews.

The public is entitled to important medical information without unreasonable delay, and editors have a responsibility to do their part in this process. Doctors need to have reports available in full detail, however, before they can advise their patients about the conclusions. In addition, media reports of scientific research before the work has been peer reviewed and fully published may lead to the dissemination of inaccurate or premature conclusions.

Editors may find the following recommendations useful as they seek to establish policies on these issues.

1) Editors can foster the orderly transmission of medical information from researchers, through peer-reviewed journals, to the public. This can be accomplished by an agreement with authors that they will not publicize their work while their manuscript is under consideration or awaiting publication, and an agreement with the media that they will not release their stories before publication in the journal, in return for which the journal will cooperate with them in preparing accurate stories (see below).

2) Very little medical research has such clear and urgently important clinical implications for the public's health that the news must be released before full publication in a journal. In such exceptional circumstances, however, appropriate authorities responsible for public health should make the decision and should be responsible for the advance dissemination of information to physicians and the media. If the author and the appropriate authorities wish to have a manuscript considered by a particular journal, the editor should be consulted before any public release. If editors accept the need for immediate release, they should waive their policies limiting pre-publication publicity.

3) Policies designed to limit pre-publication publicity should not apply to accounts in the media of presentations at scientific meetings or to the abstracts from these meetings (see Prior and Duplication Publication). Researchers who present their work at scientific meetings should feel free to discuss their presentations with reporters, but they should be discouraged from offering more detail about their study than was presented in their talk.

4) When an article is soon to be published, editors may wish to help the media prepare accurate reports by providing news releases, answering questions, supplying advance copies of the journal, and referring reporters to the appropriate experts. This assistance should be contingent upon the cooperation of the media in timing their release of stories to coincide with the publication of the article.

(Approved 1993)

in their presentations. In what may be an overinterpretation of journals' policies, some scientists have objected to giving talks when journalists are present, for fear that publicity would jeopardize publication of their work in a journal of choice.

Opinion varies about limiting presentation of research results in the popular media before they appear in journals. Opponents say that journalists and researchers should be allowed to exercise their own judgment more. Some object that such restrictions interfere with the important task of reporting the process, rather than just the products, of biomedical research (*Medicine and the Media* 1995, 22).

Much ado has been made of embargoes and related policies, and the topic is one of which health writers should be aware. However, stories on new research constitute—and should constitute—only a fraction of health writing. And emphasis on the timing of stories should not distract from the more important issue of stories' quality.

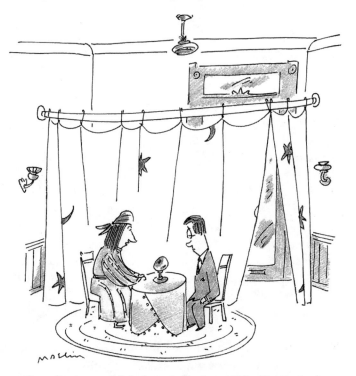

"According to an article in the upcoming issue of 'The New England Journal of Medicine,' all your fears are well founded."

Drawing by Maslin; © 1993 The New Yorker Magazine, Inc.

I. Finding Topics and Information

Searching the Journal Literature

Both for stories on new findings and for other health writing, sound background research is crucial to quality. Commonly, this background research should include obtaining previously published journal articles that pertain to the topic at hand. But how to find relevant material in the vast journal literature?

References in books can provide a start. So can those in journal articles. But in part because such references cannot be fully up to date, other searching is needed. Fortunately, the National Library of Medicine (NLM) has an extensive, readily accessible array of databases for searching the biomedical literature. The most broadly useful of these databases is MEDLINE, which contains references drawn from nearly 4,000 biomedical journals and dating back to 1966. Among other databases in this array that may aid health writers in searching the literature are AIDSLINE (regarding AIDS), BIOETHICSLINE (in biomedical ethics), HealthSTAR (in health services, technology, and administration), and HISTLINE (in history of medicine).

Traditionally, literature indexed by the NLM has been searched largely by using *Index Medicus*—a sort of medical *Readers' Guide to Periodical Literature.* A new issue of *Index Medicus* appears each month, and after each year ends, a master set of volumes is prepared that covers the entire year. Health writers can readily find references to articles on their topics by looking under subject headings of interest. Conveniently for seeking background information, *Index Medicus* contains a section devoted specifically to review articles.

In recent years, online searching of MEDLINE and other NLM databases has become easy and widely available, largely supplanting the use of *Index Medicus.* Medical libraries have computer terminals at which users can do such searching. Though protocols for searching vary, they tend to be easy to learn. And medical librarians generally are eager to introduce new users to searching and to help experienced users with especially challenging searches. If the medical library that you use offers sessions on online searching, attend if you can; the time invested will likely pay dividends later.

Increasingly, users can do online searching at their own desks rather than venturing to the library. If you work at an institution such as a medical school, a computer network may well permit such searching. Online searching of the medical literature also can be done through some com-

2. Books and Periodicals

mercial online services. In addition, the NLM now offers free MEDLINE searching at http://www.nlm.nih.gov/databases/freemedl.html. Help with NLM services is available at the toll-free phone number (888) FINDNLM.

But don't get too comfortable at your desk. Until everything that libraries offer becomes available online, the good health writer will keep venturing to general and medical libraries in search of ideas and information and assistance. The venture is likely to be well rewarded.

Chapter 3

GOVERNMENT, ASSOCIATIONS, AND OTHER INSTITUTIONS

It is fitting that this chapter, which offers guidance in finding and using institutional information sources, occurs in the middle of this section of the book. Institutions—including government agencies, associations, medical schools, and medical centers—are central sources of information for health writers. Through news releases and other channels, they generate many story ideas. And through other means, such as helping writers identify people to interview, they aid in gathering information for stories. Perhaps less obviously, such institutions publish many of the journals health writers consult and organize many of the conferences they cover.

Of course, information from institutions, like that from other sources, must be evaluated critically. Often, institutions provide information to health writers not only to disseminate knowledge for its own sake; other goals can include helping to attract funds for research or patient care, enhancing institutional reputation, attracting health-care consumers, and selling medical products. Awareness of such possible goals can aid the health writer in using institutional sources wisely—and can keep the health writer from merely being used.

The current chapter aims to help you use institutions wisely and efficiently as information resources. The chapter first offers general guidance in finding institutional sources and then summarizes types of assistance that institutions can often provide. Next come sections on major types of institutional sources: government agencies, associations, educational institutions, health-care facilities, and companies. The chapter ends by discussing how health writers can use one specific institutional resource—conferences—as a source of ideas and information.

Using Institutional Sources

Finding Institutional Sources

How can you find institutions providing the types of information you seek? A number of general resources can help. One is DIRLINE (Directory

I.   Finding Topics and Information

of Information Resources Online), a National Library of Medicine (NLM) database available at various libraries or through one's own computer. On the Internet, DIRLINE may be accessed at http://www.nlm.nih.gov/databases/locator.html. After you indicate the subject on which you are seeking information, DIRLINE identifies relevant resources such as organizations, government agencies, and academic institutions. DIRLINE also provides a brief description of each resource and indicates how it can be contacted. A printed guide, *Health Hotlines* (National Library of Medicine 1996), which is derived from DIRLINE lists toll-free telephone numbers of many institutional sources. Health writers may find it handy to keep this guide at their desks.

Various toll-free numbers for obtaining printed and other health information also are listed in a guide (National Health Information Center 1997) prepared by the federal National Health Information Center (NHIC), an information referral service. This guide, titled "Toll-Free Numbers for Health Information," is published back-to-back with a listing of federal health information centers and clearinghouses. Copies of this dual publication are available for a small handling fee from the NHIC, P.O. Box 1133, Washington, DC 20013-1133, telephone number (800) 336-4797 or (301) 565-4167. In addition, such information from NHIC may be accessed on the World Wide Web, at http://nhic-nt.health.org; the Web site includes a searchable database of organizations and government offices serving as health information resources. Selected toll-free telephone numbers from the NLM and NHIC guides are listed in Table 3-1.

Another handy, compact reference is the *ALA Fingertip Guide to National Health-Information Resources* (Kovacs 1995). Most of the 400-plus listings in this guide are for national associations; however, some government agencies concerned with health also are included. The guide can be purchased from the American Library Association by calling (800) 545-2433.

Larger reference works available mainly in libraries can aid in identifying a wide range of institutional health-information sources. One general guide, the *Medical and Health Information Directory* (Boyden 1994), contains listings of state, regional, national, and international organizations; pharmaceutical companies; state and federal government agencies; medical and allied health schools; U.S. and Canadian medical libraries; specialized clinics; and many other sources. The *Encyclopedia of Medical Organizations and Agencies* (Boyden 1996), which is organized by medical topic, includes listings of associations, national and state agencies, research centers, and other institutions. Other reference works, such as the *Encyclope-*

Table 3-1: Examples of Toll-Free Telephone Numbers for Health Information

Government Resources

National Institute on *Aging* Information Center	(800) 222-2225
CDC National *AIDS* Clearinghouse	(800) 458-5231
National Clearinghouse for *Alcohol and Drug* Information	(800) 729-6686
Alzheimer's Disease Education and Referral Center	(800) 438-4380
Cancer Information Service	(800) 4-CANCER
National Institute on *Deafness and Other Communication Disorders* Information Clearinghouse	(800) 241-1044
Agency for *Health Care Policy and Research* Clearinghouse	(800) 358-9295
National *Health Information* Center	(800) 336-4797
National *Highway Traffic Safety* Administration	(800) 424-9393
National *Library* of Medicine	(800) 272-4787
Medicare Telephone Hotline	(800) 638-6833
Office of *Minority Health* Resource Center	(800) 444-6472
National Institute of *Neurological Disorders and Stroke*	(800) 352-9424
Clearinghouse for *Occupational Safety and Health* Information	(800) 35-NIOSH
U.S. Consumer *Product Safety* Commission Hotline	(800) 638-2772
National *Rehabilitation* Information Center	(800) 346-2742
Rural Information Center *Health* Service	(800) 633-7701
Centers for Disease Control and Prevention Office on *Smoking* and Health	(800) CDC-1311
Centers for Disease Control and Prevention National *STD* Hotline	(800) 227-8922

Nongovernment Resources

Alzheimer's Association	(800) 272-3900
Arthritis Foundation Information Line	(800) 283-7800
Asthma Information Line (sponsored by American Academy of Allergy and Immunology)	(800) 822-2762
Asthma and Allergy Foundation of America	(800) 727-8462
National Reference Center for *Bioethics* Literature	(800) MEDETHX
American Council of the *Blind*	(800) 424-8666
American *Cancer* Society Response Line	(800) 227-2345

Table 3-1: Telephone Numbers (*continued*)

United *Cerebral Palsy* Association	(800) 872-5827
Cystic Fibrosis Foundation	(800) 344-4823
Deafness Research Foundation	(800) 535-3323
American *Diabetes* Association	(800) 232-3472
Epilepsy Foundation of America	(800) 332-1000
National *Headache* Foundation	(800) 843-2256
Hearing Helpline	(800) EAR-WELL
American *Heart* Association	(800) 242-8721
National *Kidney* Foundation	(800) 622-9010
American *Liver* Foundation	(800) 223-0179
Lupus Foundation of America	(800) 558-0121
National *Mental Health* Association	(800) 969-6642
National *Multiple Sclerosis* Society	(800) FIGHT-MS
American Dietetic Association's Consumer *Nutrition* Hotline	(800) 366-1655
United Network for *Organ Sharing*	(800) 243-6667
American *Parkinson's Disease* Association	(800) 223-2732
National *Parkinson* Foundation, Inc.	(800) 327-4545
Planned Parenthood Federation of America, Inc.	(800) 669-0156
National Organization for *Rare Disorders*	(800) 999-6673
National *Safety* Council	(800) 621-7619
Sickle Cell Disease Association of America, Inc.	(800) 421-8453
American *Speech-Language-Hearing* Association	(800) 638-8255
American Heart Association *Stroke* Connection	(800) 553-6321
National *Stroke* Association	(800) 787-6537
American *Trauma* Society	(800) 556-7890

NOTE: Governmental and nongovernmental resources are listed separately. Within each group, resources are listed alphabetically by subject area.

dia of Associations (Jaszczak 1997), which is discussed later in this chapter, provide assistance in finding institutional sources of given types. Not only can such reference works aid in finding institutional sources of information on given topics; merely browsing through them can suggest many story ideas.

Another resource useful in identifying various relevant institutions is

3. Government, Associations, Institutions

EurekAlert!, a World Wide Web site focusing on science and medical news. A portion of this site, at http://www.eurekalert.org/links/research_ instit.html, lists universities, companies, medical centers, professional societies, federal agencies, research institutes, and other institutional sources of information. Links to these institutions' Web sites are provided. Also, the American Association for the Advancement of Science periodically issues printed guides listing names and telephone numbers of contact people at various institutions; for information, contact the News and Public Information Office, American Association for the Advancement of Science, 1200 New York Avenue, NW, Washington, DC 20005, telephone (202) 326-6718.

If you do not know which person or office to contact at an institution, call the main number, explain that you are a health writer, and ask to speak with someone in public relations or media relations. Institutions' offices providing information to writers have a variety of names, including public information, public affairs, public relations, media relations, and communications. But by explaining your goal, you should be able to reach an appropriate person. If all else fails, ask to reach the office of the head of the institution; a staff member there should be able to direct you appropriately. Indeed, at sources such as small associations, the director may serve as the main media contact.

Contacting a public information professional at one institution often helps in finding those at others. Staff at various institutions concerned with the same area of health are aware of each other and, indeed, sometimes collaborate on programs. Thus, for example, a call to a government information office concerned with a given area of health may, in addition to providing information on the topic, lead you to contacts at pertinent associations and research centers. If information officers do not suggest people to contact elsewhere, feel free to ask.

And finally, Internet resources can aid in finding and contacting institutional sources. As will be discussed in Chapter 5, searching the World Wide Web can uncover institutional sources of potential interest. And viewing institutions' home pages, which sometimes offer online access to their publications, can provide information you seek and help you decide whether to pursue the source further. If obtaining further information from the source is your wish, the home page may provide an electronic mail (e-mail) address you can use to do so.

But what kinds of assistance can institutional sources provide? The next section provides an overview.

I. Finding Topics and Information

Seeking Types of Assistance

From generating story ideas to reviewing your writing for accuracy, institutional sources can help. Sometimes the mere name of an institution may suggest a topic. And particularly if you focus on a given area of health or report health news from a given locale, institutions can be ongoing sources of story ideas. If you specialize in writing about a particular area of health, arrange to receive news releases and other materials regularly from associations and other institutions in your area of focus; increasingly, such materials are becoming available by e-mail and on the World Wide Web. Also check periodically with public information staff at those institutions to help keep abreast of the field. Similarly if you write health stories with a local angle, get on the distribution lists of, and stay in touch with, public information staff at sites such as nearby health centers, health departments, and medical schools. As always, review items critically to determine whether they are indeed worthy of stories; be alert for what may be little more than ploys for publicity.

Once you have a story idea, institutional sources can provide various types of help in gathering information for stories. Commonly they have publications such as fact sheets or brochures to offer; sometimes more substantial works are available as well. Increasingly, institutions' publications are available on the World Wide Web, obviating the need to order them. Also, public information staff often can provide perspective on a topic. In addition, they can recommend people to interview—for instance, administrators, researchers, clinicians, and patients—and help arrange the interviews. Sometimes they can aid in checking whether information is accurate or suggest others to do so. More detailed examples of assistance are provided in the following sections, which discuss various categories of institutional sources.

Government

A wealth of information on health is available from federal, state, and local governments; for health writers this information represents taxes well spent. Two commercial reference works useful in identifying offices or individuals to contact are the *Federal Staff Directory* (Brownson 1996) and the *National Health Directory* (Ankrapp 1996). Also, the World Wide Web site for the U.S. Department of Health and Human Services, at http://www.os.dhhs.gov, includes phone numbers for media contacts at

3. Government, Associations, Institutions

various HHS agencies. Some government components especially valuable as idea and information sources for health writing are discussed below.

The National Institutes of Health

The mission of the National Institutes of Health (NIH) is to uncover new knowledge that will lead to better health. NIH pursues this mission by funding research at sites such as universities, by conducting research in its own laboratories, by helping to train investigators, and by fostering communication of biomedical information. The high priority that NIH places on communication makes it a particularly rich resource for health writers. As well as providing information on new research, NIH is a good source of information in areas of ongoing interest, such as health conditions and their management.

NIH—which is located in Bethesda, Maryland (a suburb of Washington, DC)—consists of more than 20 institutes, centers, and divisions. Each of these components has a public information office. Staff in these offices provide information directly to the public, for example by preparing publications and answering public inquiries, and they work with the media. Telephone numbers of NIH information offices are presented in Table 3-2.

Different components of NIH originated at different times, making the institution somewhat of an agglomeration. Some components—such as the National Heart, Lung, and Blood Institute and the National Institute of Dental Research—focus on certain body systems or parts. Some—such as the National Cancer Institute and the National Institute of Allergy and Infectious Diseases—deal with given categories of disease. Some—the National Institute of Child Health and Human Development and the National Institute on Aging—are concerned with specific periods of life. And others—such as the National Library of Medicine—have yet other emphases. Given this welter, how can health writers know where at NIH to obtain the information they seek?

Often, the name of an NIH component makes clear where to find information on a given health topic. And NIH has prepared an index listing hundreds of topics and indicating which NIH component(s) to consult for information on each. As well as being available in print (National Institutes of Health Office of Communications 1996), this index is available online, at gopher://gopher.nih.gov:70/11/clin/nih-infobook. The printed version is alphabetical, and that online is searched by keywords. If you are

Table 3-2. Telephone Numbers of NIH Public Information Offices

National Institutes of Health	*Phone Number*
National Cancer Institute (NCI)	(301) 496-6641
National Eye Institute (NEI)	(301) 496-5248
National Heart, Lung, and Blood Institute (NHLBI)	(301) 496-4236
National Human Genome Research Institute (NHGRI)	(301) 402-0911
National Institute on Aging (NIA)	(301) 496-1752
National Institute on Alcohol Abuse and Alcoholism (NIAAA)	(301) 443-3860
National Institute of Allergy and Infectious Diseases (NIAID)	(301) 402-1663
National Institute of Arthritis and Musculoskeletal and Skin Diseases (NIAMS)	(301) 496-8188
National Institute of Child Health and Human Development (NICHD)	(301) 496-5133
National Institute on Deafness and Other Communication Disorders (NIDCD)	(301) 496-7243
National Institute of Dental Research (NIDR)	(301) 496-4261
National Institute of Diabetes and Digestive and Kidney Diseases (NIDDK)	(301) 496-3583
National Institute on Drug Abuse (NIDA)	(301) 443-1124
National Institute of Environmental Health Sciences (NIEHS)	(919) 541-3345
National Institute of General Medical Sciences (NIGMS)	(301) 496-7301
National Institute of Mental Health (NIMH)	(301) 443-4536
National Institute of Neurological Disorders and Stroke (NINDS)	(301) 496-5924
National Institute of Nursing Research (NINR)	(301) 496-0207
Selected Other Components	
National Library of Medicine (NLM)	(301) 496-6308
Office of Alternative Medicine (OAM)	(301) 496-1712
Office of Medical Applications of Research (OMAR)	(301) 496-1144

NOTE: The home pages of various NIH components can be accessed through the NIH home page, at http://www.nih.gov.

stumped and lack access to this index, call the main NIH telephone number, (301) 496-4000; the NIH telephone operators are trained to direct callers to the appropriate information offices. Because some health topics are addressed by more than one NIH component, the first information office you contact may also direct you to others.

You can often use your time and that of NIH staff most efficiently by beginning your NIH information search via the World Wide Web. Starting at the NIH home page (http://www.nih.gov), you can access various types of information and reach the home pages of specific NIH components. These home pages, in turn, commonly provide online access to items of use to health writers—for example, news releases, lists of brochures and other publications, and instructions for ordering publications; sometimes the full text of a publication is displayed. Not only can the NIH Web site aid in background research. Also, if you seek story ideas, consider scanning the Web site with a particular eye to material highlighted as new.

Staff members at NIH information offices can give you assistance well beyond that available on the Web. Often highly experienced providing information in their fields, they can help supply the perspective needed for good health writing; for example, if you inquire about a given piece of research, they may also identify related studies. And they can be a good source of suggestions of people to interview. Among sources they may suggest are researchers at NIH, researchers elsewhere whose work is funded by NIH, and NIH administrators well situated to summarize and comment on research done at various sites. Information specialists at NIH also may direct you to other government agencies and to nongovernmental organizations that can provide information. And of course they may supply you with NIH publications you have not yet obtained through other routes.

NIH and health writers have a mission in common. Become familiar with NIH, and make good use of this resource. Quite likely, it will facilitate and strengthen your work.

Other Federal Components

Although other federal components concerned with health tend to be oriented less than NIH to disseminating information or to have fewer resources to do so, they can also be valuable resources for health writers. And of course for news reporters covering health, material from these institutions can be important to cover. Among these institutions are the Centers for Disease Control and Prevention (CDC) and the Food and Drug Administration (FDA). Both institutions, like NIH, are parts of the Department of Health and Human Services.

Located in Atlanta, Georgia, CDC has the mission: "to promote health and quality of life by preventing and controlling disease, injury, and disability." Among its components are the National Center for Chronic Disease Prevention and Health Promotion; the National Center for Environmental Health; the National Center for Health Statistics; the National Center for HIV, STD, and TB Prevention; the National Center for Infectious Diseases; the National Center for Injury Prevention and Control; and the National Institute for Occupational Safety and Health. On invitation, staff from CDC work with state and local health personnel to investigate outbreaks of disease. CDC also publishes the *Morbidity and Mortality Weekly Report,* noted earlier as a source of story ideas and information.

The CDC home page (http://www.cdc.gov) offers access to various types of information, including news releases. In addition, CDC has an automated fax information service available by telephone 24 hours a day throughout the year. Fact sheets and other documents on various diseases and other health topics may be ordered; they are immediately transmitted by fax. For this service, call (404) 332-4565. A similar service that provides pre-recorded telephone messages is available by calling (404) 332-4555. Also, the CDC media relations office can be contacted by phone at (404) 639-3286 and by fax at (404) 639-7394.

Unlike NIH and CDC, the FDA is a regulatory agency. Drugs and medical devices require FDA approval in order to be marketed in the United States; this approval is granted based on evidence of safety and effectiveness. Once drugs and medical devices enter the market, the FDA continues to monitor them. The FDA also monitors the safety and wholesomeness of food and sets standards for its labeling. In addition, it oversees the safety of such items as vaccines, cosmetics, radiation-emitting products, and the blood supply. The FDA is headquartered in Rockville, Maryland, near Washington, DC.

The FDA home page (http://www.fda.gov) provides online access to news releases and fact sheets as well as other information. Additional assistance is available from the press office at FDA headquarters. To contact this office, print reporters should call (301) 827-6242, TV and radio reporters (301) 827-3434. The public affairs specialists at FDA district offices are also a resource for health writers (Adams and Henkel 1995); to contact such an office, consult the telephone directory of the nearest large city

3. Government, Associations, Institutions

(turn to the United States government listings, and look for the FDA under "Health and Human Services").

Though smaller, another federal component that can aid the health writer is the Office of Disease Prevention and Health Promotion (ODPHP), which includes the National Health Information Center (NHIC), a health information referral service. ODPHP is in Washington, DC; its public-affairs telephone number is (202) 205-5968. The ODPHP home page can be reached at http://odphp.osophs.dhhs.gov.

One handy publication from ODPHP is an annual calendar of "health observances"—that is, months, weeks, and days devoted to promoting particular health concerns. (Examples: American Heart Month, National Hernia Month, National Diabetes Education Week, National Safety Week, Save Your Vision Week, National Senior Health and Fitness Day, World No Tobacco Day, and National Condom Day—aptly, February 14.) For each health observance, an organization or institution that can provide information is identified. Single copies of this calendar, which can help in finding story ideas and information sources, may be obtained by calling the NHIC at (800) 336-4797. The calendar also is posted on the NHIC Web site, at http://nhic-nt.health.org.

State and Local Government

Especially if you write for local or regional media, state and local health departments (and other health-related components of state and local government) can be important sources. Working with health departments is a must when covering local outbreaks of disease. These departments also can provide statistical and other information helpful in addressing a topic from a local angle. And their programs can be good subjects for stories.

Health departments of states and larger locales commonly include public information professionals who serve as contacts with the media (Gellert et al. 1994); if possible, get to know such people when you are not under deadline pressure and they are not under the pressure of communicating in a crisis. In smaller settings, a public health official such as the health officer may be the main contact. Such individuals vary in their experience with and attitude toward the media. Thus, they are less likely than public information staff to be waiting with the information you need in the form you need it. However, advance acquaintance and mutual patience can help you to work together well.

I. Finding Topics and Information

Organizations

Think of a disease—or hear of a disease for the first time—and quite likely you can find an organization concerned specifically with it. Ditto for any health profession or subspecialty thereof. These health-related organizations have much information to provide and can suggest many topics for stories. But how can you identify such organizations? What do they have to offer? And how can you use this information source soundly?

The online health-resource database DIRLINE, the *ALA Fingertip Guide to National Health-Information Resources,* and other references discussed early in this chapter include listings of associations. And the *Encyclopedia of Associations* (Jaszczak 1997) devotes a substantial section to health and medical organizations, of which it lists more than 2,000. As well as being widely available at libraries, the *Encyclopedia of Associations* can be accessed through the online services DIALOG and NEXIS. Among types of information commonly provided on the associations listed are main purposes and activities, size of membership, size of staff, budget, subgroups, publications, dates of conventions or major meetings, address, telephone number (and, in many cases, a toll-free number), and fax number. Clearly, much of this information can aid the health writer in deciding whether, how, and for what types of information to contact given organizations.

Also, twice a year *JAMA: The Journal of the American Medical Association* publishes a several-page listing titled "Organizations of Medical Interest"; among organizations listed are associations in various medical specialties. The listing includes addresses, phone numbers, and dates of meetings. Because the listing is alphabetical rather than by topic, it is not well suited for seeking organizations to contact in search of information for a given story. However, the list can easily be scanned in search of organizations for future reference, and skimming it can yield story ideas. (What of interest, for example, might the Association for the Advancement of Automotive Medicine have to share? the Wilderness Medical Society? the American Center for Chinese Medical Sciences?) Twice a year as well, *JAMA* publishes listings of state medical associations.

Among associations that often have considerable information available to health writers are those focusing on given diseases or groups thereof. Sometimes called voluntary health organizations, these range from large organizations concerned with widespread causes of death or disability— for example, the American Heart Association, the American Cancer Society, and the Arthritis Foundation—to small groups concerned with one or another rare disease, to even the National Pediculosis (yes, that means lice

3. Government, Associations, Institutions

infestation) Association. Although different health associations differ in their mix of efforts, common and often overlapping goals include supporting research, promoting prevention, improving treatment, and educating health professionals and the public. Some of the associations also work to influence policies affecting people with given health conditions or to change attitudes toward these people. Often, voluntary health organizations are active in fundraising; before and during fund drives, they commonly seek media attention. In addition to national headquarters, many associations have local chapters, which can be good places to start seeking information.

"The associations are usually the first place I look for information," says Catherine Dold, a freelancer whose health articles have appeared in *Cosmopolitan, Living Fit, Cancer Smart,* and other publications. Because various goals of voluntary health organizations entail conveying information to the public, these organizations tend to be quite accommodating to health writers—and, indeed, to court health writers' attention. Unless such organizations are small, they commonly have staff members specializing in media relations.

Brochures and other publications typically are available on topics the association deals with; some of the larger associations have media guides or other publications designed specifically as background for health writers and other journalists. Sometimes videotaped material is available for viewing or broadcasting, and increasingly such organizations are establishing sites on the World Wide Web. (Freelancer Dold says she usually starts her information search by looking for relevant organizations' sites on the Web.) The associations commonly issue news releases; if associations publish journals, some of the releases may deal with research reported therein. News releases and related materials also are issued regarding conferences of the associations; especially at large national conferences, press briefings may be held on research being reported, and a newsroom may be available where health reporters and others covering the conference may work.

Also, some of the larger associations organize science writers' conferences or science writers' seminars to inform the media about work in their fields. When health writers seek researchers, clinicians, or patients to interview, associations provide referrals. Some associations' media offices have databases listing experts available to interview on various topics.

Associations of scientists likewise tend to offer some or all of the above. For example, an extensive array of press conferences, many of them on health-related topics, accompanies the annual meeting of the American Association for the Advancement of Science. Among other scientific societies that include many biomedical researchers and have active media programs are the American Society for Microbiology and the Society for Neuroscience.

Associations of health professionals also can assist health writers. Among such national organizations are the American Medical Association, the American Dental Association, the American Nurses Association, the American Dietetic Association, the American Occupational Therapy Association, the American Physical Therapy Association, the American Academy of Physician Assistants, and the American Veterinary Medical Association. More localized organizations such as state medical associations and county medical societies also exist, as do organizations in various medical specialties. Among resources commonly available from health-professional associations are publications on the professions they represent and the health conditions their members deal with, assistance in covering research reported in journals the associations publish or conferences they hold, and referral to members to interview on given subjects. Like other organizations, various associations in the health professions have World Wide Web sites containing information for the media and other material that can aid health writers.

Voluntary health organizations, scientific societies, and professional associations can help the health writer on both an "acute" and a "chronic" basis. Their written, human, and other resources can aid considerably in gathering information for immediate stories. And on an ongoing basis, they can aid in finding story ideas and staying up-to-date.

Like information from other resources, however, that from organizations should be evaluated critically. Is a development truly newsworthy, or might the organization largely be seeking publicity, perhaps just before a fund drive? Does a recommendation have a sound scientific basis, or could it have been generated in part to serve the association's own interests? Is a given disease worthy of considerable coverage, or does an assertive association make it seem more important than it is? Asking such questions can help you make soundest use of organizations as a source.

Educational Institutions

Good health writers are perpetual students. Although they may not enroll in classes, they often draw on educational institutions such as medical and other health-professional schools. Involved in education, research, and patient care, these schools are a substantial source of story ideas and information.

You can draw on institutions such as medical schools in various ways. Keep track of their calendars of events, and attend presentations that may yield stories or serve as useful background. Obtain their publications, and scan them for material of interest. And consult their public information offices.

Public information offices of health-professional schools can aid in finding story ideas and identifying experts to interview. If given schools, such as local medical schools, are of particular interest, check how you can best obtain their news releases in printed or electronic form. Also talk with public relations staff members, who can help you find more distinctive story ideas than those presented in news releases. As well as requesting experts to interview on given topics, check whether the school has a guide listing faculty members' areas of special expertise. Some schools provide printed guides to journalists or post such guides on the World Wide Web.

Public information professionals at educational institutions strive, of course, to promote the images of their institutions. Good professionals, however, know better than to oversell; indeed, they sometimes recommend outside sources better suited to provide given types of information. Nevertheless, the need to evaluate information for newsworthiness and other value remains for this source as for others.

Health-Care Institutions

Hospitals, clinics, and other health-care institutions can be sources of doctors and other experts to interview. And sometimes new programs or services that they offer are worthy of stories. Here too, public relations staff can aid you. Here too, work with them toward your mutual goals but also retain your own judgment.

Industry

Like educational and health-care institutions, pharmaceutical companies and manufacturers of medical devices have public relations offices. These offices commonly have considerable material to offer regarding the companies' products. Some also have materials available regarding conditions for which their products are intended. One handy resource for identifying public relations contact people at pharmaceutical companies is the annual *Reporter's Handbook for the Prescription Drug Industry* (PhRMA 1996), available to journalists from the Pharmaceutical Research and Manufacturers of America, phone (202) 835-3400. Draw on companies as resources, but of course keep in mind their commercial interests.

Conferences

Many institutions such as those noted in this chapter, hold conferences dealing with health. For example, NIH holds *consensus conferences* to evaluate and integrate information on items such as health care technologies. And various health-related organizations have annual meetings. Whether you actually attend or not, conferences can provide you with many story ideas and much information.

How can you find out about conferences that may be of interest? Some guides discussed earlier in this chapter—for example, the *Encyclopedia of Associations*—include conference dates for institutions listed; the organizations can then be contacted for further information. Twice a year *JAMA* publishes a list of upcoming meetings in the United States, and twice a year it publishes a list of such meetings abroad. Some other journals also publish announcements of conferences. Lists of meetings also are available on the Web, for example at http://www.lib.uwaterloo.ca/society/meetings.html. After the fact, you can read about conference highlights in sites such as *Science News,* the news sections of *Science* and *JAMA,* and news periodicals for health professionals.

Few health writers have the funding and time to attend many conferences, but benefits can be obtained even from those not attended. Looking at conference programs can suggest story ideas to pursue and experts to consult. Often, written materials from conferences—news releases, media backgrounders, abstracts or texts of presentations, and written recommendations issued—are available from the public information office of the group holding the conference; audiotapes sometimes can be obtained as well.

When you do attend a conference, how can you make best use of the time and other resources invested? The following tips can be of help:

• Find out about media registration. As a health writer, you may be able to attend the conference free. You also may receive materials in advance that can help you prepare. If seeking media registration, be ready to offer

3. Government, Associations, Institutions

proof that you either work for the media, have a freelance assignment to cover the conference, or belong to a professional organization such as the National Association of Science Writers.

• Review the conference program carefully in advance. Large conferences often include many simultaneous sessions. To choose most soundly among them, spend some time checking the program beforehand.

• Consider doing some background research. As emphasized repeatedly in this book, good health writing includes context. If you must submit a story shortly after a presentation, try to do background research in advance. For example, read up on the topic; find out about related work; perhaps even interview the presenter in advance if doing so may not be feasible at the conference.

• Make good use of resources provided for the media. At many conferences, written materials on the sessions are available for reporters to take, public information staff are on hand to aid in such tasks as arranging interviews, and space is available in which to work. Sometimes news conferences also are held. Find out about such resources, and make use of them.

• Obtain material for both immediate and long-term use. As well as looking for immediate stories, be alert for items to consider using in future projects. Also be on the lookout for possible trends to keep watching. Be prepared to carry home lots of material for potential long-term use.

• Recognize that research findings reported at conferences may be preliminary or largely unreviewed. To be accepted for presentation at a conference, research generally need not pass nearly as stringent or detailed review as to be published in a journal. Thus, much of the research presented at a conference may be preliminary or of limited quality. If research still appears exploratory, make that fact clear in your writing, if you cover the research at all. Also think carefully about whether research is strong enough to merit reporting. (For assistance in assessing research strength, see Chapter 6.)

• Make note of speakers to consider interviewing in the future. Conferences serve in part as showcases for experts. You can see which ones appear approachable and express themselves clearly and engagingly. And you can discern which ones seem likely to come across well in the broadcast media. If a speaker seems particularly well suited for interviews, take note for future use.

• Consider teaming up with another health writer to gather materials and information. Even the most resourceful health writer can be in only one place at once. If more than one session at a given time is of interest, consider trading notes and handouts with a colleague.

• Take advantage of the news room as a place to network. News rooms at conferences provide opportunity to talk with fellow health writers from various media and public relations settings. They are good places to learn of job openings, to find out about resources, and to discuss issues of professional concern. Ultimately, time spent informally in the newsroom may be some of your most productive time at a conference.

• Shortly after the conference, review and organize the material obtained. On returning from a conference, you may face pressure to deal immediately with all that is waiting; you may also be tempted merely to collapse. However, do not just dump your conference materials in a corner. Rather, while memories of the conference are still fresh, review and clarify your notes. Also file the materials you obtained in a way that allows you to draw on them productively.

• Consider thanking public relations staff who aided in your coverage of the conference. Too often, these professionals receive feedback only when something goes wrong. When assistance such as that at a conference goes particularly right, take a moment to convey your thanks. A few words in person, a brief e-mail message, or a thanks-bearing copy of a resulting story is all it takes. As well as being professional and polite, such courtesy can facilitate continuing to draw on institutional sources—some of the health writer's main resources for ideas and information.

Chapter 4

RESEARCHERS, CLINICIANS, PATIENTS, AND OTHERS

You've reviewed the literature on your topic. You've gathered information from relevant institutions. In doing so, quite likely you have drawn on some of the newest information technologies. But do not neglect one of the oldest—talking with people who have pertinent expertise and experience.

For the health writer, interviewing is crucial in gathering information and generating new story ideas. It lets you learn about the latest work. It lets you check on items that are unclear. It allows access to expert opinion. It lets you learn about the process, not just the products, of biomedical research. It lets you explore the human side of being a researcher, a health professional, or someone affected by an illness. It also can provide a local angle. For print media, it supplies the quotes and anecdotes that help make health writing engaging. For broadcast, it supplies voices and human visuals important to a piece.

This chapter focuses on human sources: researchers, clinicians, patients, and others. It begins with guidance on finding appropriate people to interview. Next it addresses deciding on the interview medium and doing the interview. Finally, it discusses various major groups of sources and provides suggestions for working with them.

Identifying People to Interview

In gathering information thus far for your story, you almost certainly have identified people to consider interviewing. Your reading quite likely has disclosed authors to contact for further information on their work or to consult more broadly. And your contacts with associations and institutions probably have yielded suggestions of people to talk with. Two additional resources can help you round out your list of interview candidates.

One resource is the Media Resource Service (MRS). This free service, which started in 1980, provides journalists with referrals to scientists, physicians, policy makers, and others who have expertise in given areas relating to science and have agreed to provide information to the media. In making referrals, the MRS staff draws on a database of about 30,000 experts, many of them in biomedical fields; if an area is controversial, the staff identifies experts with a representative range of views. Formerly a program of the Scientists' Institute for Public Information, the MRS currently is sponsored by the scientific research society Sigma Xi. It is funded by contributions from various media companies, other corporations, and foundations. The MRS can be reached by telephone at (800) 223-1730 or (919) 547-5240, by fax at (919) 549-0090, and by e-mail at mediaresource@ sigmaxi.org. Contacting the MRS by telephone tends to be best because staff can immediately ask questions to clarify your needs.

Alan McGowan, president of the MRS, has offered the following advice about using this resource: If possible, avoid waiting until the last minute to call. Describe the story you are working on, and be specific about the area in which you are seeking expertise. To avoid duplication, indicate which experts you already have contacted or plan to contact. Also, if you are calling the MRS for the first time, be ready to describe your background; this information aids the staff in recommending experts well suited to provide information at an appropriate level.

Another resource is ProfNet, the Professors Network, services of which include aid in finding expert sources. ProfNet links members of the media to public information officers at universities, medical centers, government agencies, and other sites via the Internet. When a health writer or other journalist submits an information request or query to ProfNet, it is distributed to the public information officers at the member institutions; these individuals can then recommend experts to consult.

If you use ProfNet to seek expert sources, your query should state your name, the publication for which you are writing, the nature of your project, the type of expertise or information sought, the time frame within which you are working, and the way that public information officers should contact you. If possible, provide at least two of the following: your telephone number, your fax number, and your e-mail address. Queries can be submitted by e-mail to profnet@profnet.com, by fax to (516) 689-1425, and by phone to (800) PROFNET. Further information about ProfNet is available on the World Wide Web at http://www.profnet.com.

As you gain experience as a health writer, you probably will develop your own group of favorite sources in various fields—people who are knowledgeable, articulate, and ready to talk. Make good use of these sources but do not overuse them, as some health writers tend to do. The health community is a large one; let many voices be heard.

4.   Researchers, Clinicians, Patients, Others

Tips on Interviewing

In addition to whom you interview, how you interview affects what you learn. The following tips on interviewing are geared particularly to health writers. For the health writer without a journalism background, additional guidance is available in the near-classic *The Craft of Interviewing* (Brady 1976), more recent guides to interviewing, such as *Interviews That Work* (Biagi 1992), and basic journalism textbooks. Health writers with backgrounds in the health professions may find the principles of interviewing sources much like those of interviewing patients.

Deciding on the Interview Medium

Consider the best medium for the interview. Many health writers depend largely on interviewing by telephone. This medium can make efficient use of time, and of course it is well suited for interviewing people far away. Also, sometimes patients who are sensitive about their health conditions feel more comfortable being interviewed by telephone than face-to-face. Consider, however, written formats and especially interviews in person as alternatives to the telephone. Although written media, such as e-mail, do not permit as spontaneous an interchange as a spoken interview does, they can work well for gaining answers to straightforward questions, for example, before or after a more traditional interview. And e-mail or other written formats can be a good choice for interviewing people who have difficulty hearing or speaking.

If circumstances permit, try to do major interviews in person. In person you can gain information unavailable otherwise. You can note people's appearances and observe their expressions; the nonverbal cues you perceive can aid in directing the interview. You also can see what a given laboratory, clinic, or other facility looks like; your observations may prompt questions, and you may be able to tour the facility. If you interview someone with a health condition, doing so in the person's home or office may help you more readily see how the condition has (or has not) affected the person's life.

Being present in person also facilitates talking with colleagues, family members, or others close to the person being interviewed or doing related work. It can aid in obtaining written materials that can help with your story, as well as in thinking of visuals to accompany it. In short, interviewing in person can yield various insights, materials, and details that can strengthen your health writing.

Preparing, Interviewing, and Following Up

Before the interview, brief yourself well. (Don't be like the reporter who turned to her neighbor at a news conference and whispered, "I've heard about those 'kidney things,' now what do they do?") Review the reading you have done and any other material you have obtained. Develop a list of questions in advance, but remain flexible to pursue unexpected leads. Resist the temptation to flaunt the knowledge you have gathered; remember, as an interviewer your main task is to listen.

During the interview, be a good listener. Do not rush in with a comment or new question if the person you are interviewing hesitates; give the person sufficient time to think. If answers are unclear, do request clarification. And to check your understanding and elicit elaboration, restate in your own words what you understood the source to say. Near the end of the interview, check whether the source has anything to add; often doing so yields important material for the story or ideas for additional stories. If some questions may be sensitive, save them for last.

After the interview, review your notes promptly. Read and clarify what you have written. If you also tape-recorded the interview, check the tape and transcribe material of interest. Also check with the source about any important points that are unclear; for quick checks on items such as numbers and definitions, e-mail can be handy. A good source will appreciate your care—and, more important, your readers will benefit.

Answering Requests to Review the Story

When approached for an interview, or even after the interview ends, researchers and others sometimes demand to approve the story before it is aired or printed. Obtaining such approval, even when not explicitly requested, is common in public relations settings. For example, after drafting a news release, a health writer at a university normally shows it to the researcher whose work is being described. If the researcher is uncomfortable with anything in it, the writer works to come up with a version that is acceptable to the researcher and still effectively fulfills a release's functions.

Reporters' and freelancers' stories for the media are not subject to such review; the writers and editors have the final say. However, as discussed in Chapter 7, asking those interviewed to check relevant passages for technical accuracy can be prudent practice. Often, assurance of a chance to do so will allay a source's concerns. And, if it is clear from the interview that the health writer is well prepared and attentive to detail, sources will likely feel much less need to have tight control.

Interviewing Members of Various Groups

Though similar interviewing skills can aid in interviewing anyone from a child with a disease to the discoverer of a newly found gene, types of sources differ somewhat in how they are best approached. How can you best locate sources of various types? What attitudes toward the media do they tend to bring to the interview? How can you best work with such sources? The following sections address such questions.

Researchers

Biomedical researchers to interview can be identified in various ways. Authors of journal articles are obvious candidates, as are speakers at conferences. In addition, public information staff at government agencies, associations, and universities can suggest researchers to interview. And the Media Resource Service and ProfNet are well geared to identify researchers.

Background information on a researcher can help you decide what to ask, as well as adding to an article itself. Various sources of such information exist. *American Men and Women of Science* (1994) provides basic biographical data on many prominent scientists; also, many scientists are listed in biographical guides such as *Who's Who*. Public information staff at researchers' institutions often can provide biographical information, and many researchers have home pages on the World Wide Web. Of course, you can ask a researcher for a copy of his or her curriculum vitae (essentially the academic equivalent of a resume).

Researchers vary in their attitudes toward the media; often a given researcher has mixed views. On the one hand, researchers voice various objections to dealing with the press. Some say that their work is too technical for the public to understand, that they lack the time to talk with reporters, that colleagues would criticize them for seeming to seek publicity, or that talking with the media about their work would jeopardize their chances of publishing it in a journal; some have had bad experiences or have heard of them and say, "never again" (Rodgers and Adams 1994). On the other hand, some researchers seek publicity; motives include bolstering the reputation of their research field or of science in general, enhancing the image of their institution, helping to attract funding, advancing causes that they support, or enhancing their egos. Also, researchers vary considerably in their experience working with reporters. Some are extremely media-savvy, others are largely unacquainted with how the media work.

A study of researchers who had published articles in *JAMA* or the *New England Journal of Medicine* found generally positive attitudes toward the press (Wilkes and Kravitz 1992). More than 60 percent of the respondents agreed that media coverage helps inform the professional community of their research. Indeed, research over the years supports the view that, in addition to informing the public, stories in the popular media increase health professionals' and researchers' awareness of developments in their fields (Shaw and Van Nevel 1967; Phillips et al. 1991).

"Experts (particularly the ones who might be getting a flurry of atten-

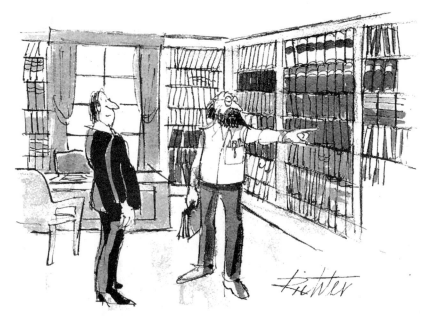

"On that shelf are my scholarly books. On that shelf are journals in which my scholarly articles have appeared, and on that shelf are video and audio tapes of my appearances on talk shows."

Cartoon © Mischa Richter and Harald Bakken, for the *Chronicle of Higher Education.*

tion because of a paper or controversy) have busy schedules," a public information staffer at a medical school notes. As well as doing their research, they must publish journal articles about it if they are to maintain their careers. In most settings, they also must write grant proposals seeking funding for their research—a stressful and time-consuming process. Many also teach students or see patients or both. And, they typically are involved in various other endeavors, such as evaluating manuscripts submitted to journals, speaking at conferences, and participating in professional societies.

Thus, health writers sensitive to researchers' time constraints are likely to work best with these sources. If you can, try to contact researchers well before your deadline; be flexible in scheduling interviews. To make efficient use of the interview time, consider faxing or e-mailing questions beforehand.

Most important, prepare thoroughly in advance, so researchers need not spend much time explaining basics. "My experience is that people at the top of their profession are very kind and generally pretty good at explaining complex issues if they see that you are trying to understand what they are saying," says Elizabeth Ban, for many years a medical writer for the Voice of America. "If they see you haven't done your homework, they will not give you the time of day, which is fine. You should always do your homework."

Some researchers are founts of good quotes, crisp sound bites, and nice analogies. Others, however, tend to present material in a technical and dry manner. Sometimes acting less informed than you are can elicit a simple, punchy explanation well suited to quote or to broadcast. Another tack is to ask researchers to present the material as they would to bright adolescents.

Biomedical researchers are intelligent and resourceful people, and most are highly committed to the public's health. Meet them halfway by understanding their constraints and making clear your needs. The information and ideas they provide in return can add much to your writing.

Health Professionals

Health professionals are the people most quoted and mentioned in newspaper articles about medicine or health care (Stempel and Culbertson 1984; Buresh, Gordon, and Bell 1991). They also are major information sources for health writing in other media. Interviewing them can help make your writing more informative, engaging, and authoritative.

I. Finding Topics and Information

Members of various health professions can be well worth interviewing. Traditionally, physicians have been by far the most common sources; given their expertise and leading role, they remain important interview subjects. Today, however, health care is more and more a team endeavor. And various members of the team have knowledge and communication skills that can make them excellent sources. Among the many health professionals to consider talking with are physician assistants, nurses, pharmacists, dietitians, physical therapists, and occupational therapists. Because such individuals often are less rushed than physicians (or at least have hours that are more regular), and because they often focus on patient education, they can be particularly accessible resources, both literally and figuratively.

Health professionals to interview can be identified in various ways. The public relations offices of medical schools and other health professional schools can suggest experts to interview on given topics, as can such offices at hospitals and clinics. Professional societies—national, state, and local—can suggest members with requisite expertise. Some, such as the American Nurses Association, maintain databases of members with expertise on various topics. National and local offices of voluntary health associations, such as the American Heart Association and the American Cancer Society, also can recommend health professionals to interview on given topics. Contacting such an organization can help you find knowledgeable people from various health professions.

Awareness of what physicians in various specialties do can aid in knowing what information to seek from whom. One resource in this regard is the brochure *Which Medical Specialist for You* (American Board of Medical Specialties 1995), available from the American Board of Medical Specialties (ABMS), 1007 Church Street, Suite 404, Evanston, Illinois 60201-5913, telephone (847) 491-9091. Biographical information on physicians certified in their specialties can be obtained from *The Official ABMS Directory of Board Certified Medical Specialists* (1997), found in general and medical libraries.

Various health professions and niches within them can be good topics for stories. Also, story ideas can be obtained by consulting associations in various health professions about developments in those professions.

Health professionals vary considerably in their attitudes toward the media. Some shun any contact with reporters; others avidly seek publicity, sometimes with the help of public relations consultants. Likewise, health professionals vary considerably in their awareness of how the media function and what health writers are likely to find useful.

4. Researchers, Clinicians, Patients, Others

Much of the literature on the relationship between health professionals and the media focuses on physicians. Reading this literature reveals that interaction between physicians and journalists has changed considerably in some respects over the years but that many of the issues stay the same. For example, a report on a series of meetings between doctors and reporters during the 1950s indicates that the medical profession showed great aversion at the time toward anything that could be construed as a physician seeming to seek publicity; thus it was noted that physicians often checked with their county medical societies before agreeing to speak with reporters. Yet many of the issues addressed in the meeting were the same as today. For example, participants discussed what degree of accuracy is acceptable in media reports, whether the role of the media is to educate or to inform, and whether reporters were qualified to present medical findings in adequate context (Krieghbaum 1957).

Results of a survey in the early 1990s suggest that physicians no longer consider their colleagues in the news merely publicity-seekers. However, they tend to view medical coverage in the media as being biased against physicians and the medical profession, containing technical inaccuracies, being sensationalistic, focusing too much on trendy diseases, being prone to the reporter's biases, and telling only a small part of the story. The introduction to the report in which the survey is presented emphasizes, however, that physicians and journalists share the mission of serving the public (Rubin and Rogers 1994).

In talking with health professionals, make clear your commitment to this mutual goal and your dedication to accuracy. Find out your sources' schedules and be ready to work within them; surgeons, for example, tend to start operating early in the morning but to be more available later in the day. Realize that emergencies can arise, so have back-up plans; do not wait to speak with a given source until it would be too late to contact anyone else. If health professionals lapse into technical jargon, consider suggesting that they present the material as they would to a patient. And if you are a health writer who is a health professional as well, resist the temptation to engage only in professional discussion; remember that the goal is to obtain material that will strengthen your story.

Patients

Patients—and ways to keep from becoming a patient—are what health writing is largely about. Interviewing patients and those near them can provide important perspectives and much human interest.

I. Finding Topics and Information

How can you find patients to interview? (Or both more broadly and more precisely, given that only people who are receiving medical care are rightly termed patients, how can you find people to interview who have a given condition?) One way to start is with your own acquaintances. If a condition is common, you may well know someone with it. Another way is to contact physicians, dentists, or other appropriate clinicians. Because they must maintain confidentiality, clinicians will not immediately suggest patients to contact. They may, however, let patients know that you are seeking people to interview. A third approach is to contact local or national offices of associations dealing with the condition of interest. Often, associations have available people with the condition who have indicated their willingness to be interviewed. Be aware, however, that those active in such associations or participating in support groups they sponsor may not be representative of those with a condition. For example, they may tend to be especially severely affected or attach particularly strong weight to their condition.

Indeed, given that many diseases vary widely in severity, an issue to consider is which individuals to feature in your writing. Although those most dramatically affected may make the most compelling reading, featuring only such patients conveys a distorted picture. Ideally, if articles on given diseases depict patients, they should include those affected to various extents. Just portraying someone with a severe case of a disease and stating that most cases are much milder is unlikely to suffice; those encountering the story are likely to remember the vivid case and forget the general statement.

Another issue is that of anonymity. Journalists generally try to avoid citing anonymous sources. However, there's a difference between someone claiming anonymously that the mayor is stealing public funds and someone willing to discuss personal details of an illness but unwilling to have his or her name appear in a story. In writing about health matters that may be sensitive, it generally is acceptable to maintain the source's anonymity—for example, by identifying the person only by age and profession or indicating that a name other than the person's real one is being used. The person's identity is not the point; the person's experience and perceptions are.

Although some patients, such as those who are spokespersons for organizations, are experienced in talking with journalists, many patients whom you may interview are not. In the latter case, take care to set the source at ease, to keep from raising unrealistic expectations, and to avoid abusing trust. Begin with some general conversation and basic questions about the source. Make clear the scope of your project; otherwise, patients being interviewed for a general story on a condition may assume that a story will be solely about them. Likewise, note that only a small part of the interview may appear in the final story.

If you are an attentive, empathetic listener, often the person will tell you things you might not have dared to ask. Technically, anything a source tells you is fair game to use in a story unless the source has indicated otherwise beforehand. However, a patient you interview may view you as a friend and assume you would not, for instance, include anything that would be hurtful to a family member. Consider whether such items are worth including—or whether, for example, it would suffice to say that some patients feel a given way. If in doubt, check with the person you interviewed.

Talking with patients provides important perspective on how medical conditions affect people's lives. Also, many patients are highly informed about their diseases, so interviewing them can suggest biomedical areas to explore. Realize, however, that patients may be misinformed about medical subjects or may have misheard what health professionals told them. For example, a woman with binaural (in both ears) hearing loss thought she had been told that the hearing loss was "bineural." As elsewhere in your research, cross-check your information.

Others

Not only patients but also those close to them can provide perspective. Thus, consider talking with people such as family members, close friends, and colleagues. Before approaching such sources, seek the patient's approval unless the patient is incompetent to give it.

The type of story you are preparing, and the background research you do, may also suggest people to interview other than those in groups discussed in this chapter. Among the many possibilities are social workers, medical ethicists, hospital administrators, policy makers, research administrators, and company executives. Whatever the source, do your homework first; ask and listen and listen some more; review your notes; and obtain needed clarification. Your health writing will benefit from your human sources.

Chapter 5

ONLINE RESOURCES

"I'll put something in the mail" was long a standard response when health writers called public information offices for background materials. Now, however, one increasingly hears, "Do you have access to the World Wide Web? Let me direct you to our home page." Likewise, much of what health writers did by letter or telephone is now being done by e-mail. As well as supplying old types of information in new ways, online capabilities are providing new and increased opportunities to find story ideas and information.

As may be clear from the "http's" and such scattered through the previous chapters, using the World Wide Web and other online resources has become valuable—indeed, often integral—to the health writer's work. This brief chapter focuses on these resources. The chapter assumes some basic familiarity with the Internet. And given how rapidly the Internet is changing, it emphasizes principles rather than details.

If you are unfamiliar with the Internet or seeking an update, various guides to the Internet are available. Two especially well suited for health writers are *The Online Journalist* (Reddick and King 1997) and *Computer Assisted Research: A Guide for Tapping Online Information* (Paul 1995); the latter, published by the Poynter Institute for Media Studies, may be accessed online at http://www.nando.net/prof/poynter/chome.html or ordered from the Poynter Institute, telephone (813) 821-9494. Also, general and medical librarians, who are increasingly becoming specialists in computerized as well as printed resources, can help acquaint you with online resources that suit your needs and keep you up-to-date. And libraries commonly give sessions about online resources they offer.

Introductions and updates geared specifically to using online resources in writing about health and science are available via conferences and periodicals of groups such as the American Medical Writers Association and the National Association of Science Writers. Consumer-oriented guides that health writers can draw on include *Dr. Tom Linden's Guide to Online Medicine* (Linden and Kienholz 1995), *The Internet Health, Fitness, and Medicine Yellow Pages*

I. Finding Topics and Information

(Naythons and Catsimatides 1995), and *Health Online* (Ferguson 1996). Although such books cannot be fully up-to-date, they can serve as useful starting points. And as will be discussed below, directories of online medical resources also appear, not surprisingly, online.

The World Wide Web

It is easy to get tangled up in the World Wide Web. So much material of such varied quality is present. Nearly anyone can post nearly anything online; no evidence of the information's soundness is needed. Although some Web sites have stringent requirements for material posted, the Web is hardly a peer-reviewed journal—or even a well-ordered reading room with material carefully chosen by librarians.

Fortunately, librarians and others have developed Web sites that serve as indexes to online medical offerings. Some of these indexes, "nodes," or "hubs" are listed at the top of Table 5-1. In addition, the Argus Clearinghouse, at http://www.clearinghouse.net, includes guides to Web sites in health and medicine. As a health writer, you can facilitate future searches by bookmarking some of these overarching sites.

Such indexes or hubs can lead you to a wide array of medically related sites—for journals, government agencies, professional societies, voluntary health associations, and more. Some examples of Web sites that health writers may find useful are listed in Table 5-1.

Although material obtained from the Web can be extremely useful, it should be carefully assessed. Some Web sites are of questionable validity at best or have a commercial aim; thus, let the browser beware. Consider whether the Web site is that of a highly reputable entity. If in doubt, check the information for consistency with that in sources that you trust, or confirm it through interviews with experts.

Also make sure that the information is up-to-date. Look for a date of posting or revision. If the material may be outdated, contact the source to ascertain its currency.

And finally, realize that wandering the Web can be hypnotic, and one can easily find hours gone with relatively little yield. Make good use of the Web. It can be a fine source of story ideas and background for health writing and can also lead you to sources to contact. But unless you have the time to do so, do not let browsing the Web be an end in itself.

Table 5-1:   Some Internet Sites of Potential Use to Health Writers

Medical "Hubs"
  American Medical Association (http://www.ama-assn.org)
  Medical Matrix (http://www.medmatrix.org/index.asp)
  MedWeb (http://www.emory.edu/WHSCL/medweb.html)
  Yahoo—Health (http://www.yahoo.com/Health)

Journals, etc.
  BMJ: British Medical Journal (http://www.bmj.com/bmj)
  JAMA (http://www.ama-assn.org)
  Free MEDLINE (http://www.nlm.nih.gov/databases/freemedl.html)
  The Merck Manual (http://www.merck.com)
  New England Journal of Medicine (http://www.nejm.org)
  Science (http://www.sciencemag.org)
  Science News (http://www.sciencenews.org)

Government
  Centers for Disease Control and Prevention (http://www.cdc.gov)
  Food and Drug Administration (http://www.fda.gov)
  Health Care Financing Administration (http://www.hcfa.gov)
  healthfinder™ (http://www.healthfinder.gov)
  Office of Disease Prevention and Health Promotion
      (http://odphp.osophs.dhhs.gov)
  National Health Information Center (http://nhic-nt.health.org)
  National Institutes of Health (http://www.nih.gov)
  National Library of Medicine (http://www.nlm.nih.gov)

Organizations
  American Association for the Advancement of Science
      (http://www.aaas.org)
  American Cancer Society (http://www.cancer.org)
  American Heart Association (http://www.amhrt.org)
  American Lung Association (http://www.lungusa.org)
  American Medical Association (http://www.ama-assn.org)
  American Society for Microbiology (http://www.asmusa.org)
  Arthritis Foundation (http://www.arthritis.org)
  Association of American Medical Colleges (http://www.aamc.org)
  World Health Organization (http://www.who.ch)

Sites for Journalists
  EurekAlert! (http://www.eurekalert.org)
  FACSNET (http://www.facsnet.org)
  National Association of Science Writers (http://www.nasw.org)
  ProfNet (http://www.profnet.com)
  Society of Environmental Journalists (http://www.sej.org)

I. Finding Topics and Information

Electronic Mail

For many health writers, e-mail has become as basic as the telephone. Uses include receiving materials such as news releases, setting up interviews, corresponding with editors, and taking part in online discussion groups (Morton 1996). E-mail also is handy for checking facts, and sometimes it is used for interviews.

A health writer who had recently moved to Australia found local experts unwilling to be interviewed for an important story she was doing on medical research. Using e-mail to the United States, she contacted the leading researcher in the field. "How did you get him to talk to you?" the editor of the publication marveled. "I just e-mailed him my query" was the writer's reply.

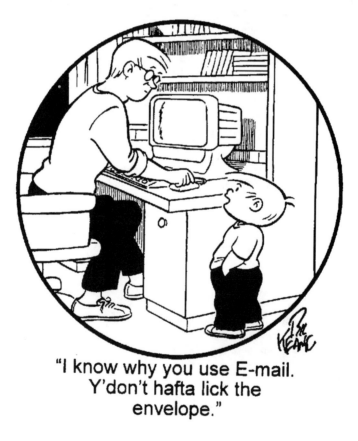

"I know why you use E-mail. Y'don't hafta lick the envelope."

5.   Online Resources

When journalist John Crewdson of the *Chicago Tribune* was preparing a series on in-flight medical emergencies, he placed a classified advertisement in the *New England Journal of Medicine* asking to hear from health professionals who had been involved in such situations. "I tossed in my e-mail address as an afterthought, but it was a good idea," recalls Crewdson, who received many replies soon after the ad appeared. "Why should anyone go to the trouble of licking a stamp and putting an envelope in a mailbox when they can do it all in front of their computer?"

Some caveats about e-mail are in order. Normal e-mail is not completely private, and it is easy to copy and forward. Thus, it is not suited for confidential material, be it a story idea you wish to hide from competitors or information on identities of patients who will be anonymous in a story. One rule of thumb: If you wouldn't send it by postcard, you probably shouldn't do so by e-mail.

Only with the consent of the sender should you include in your writing material obtained by e-mail. If the material clearly was requested for use in a story, then clearly using it is fair game. But what was offered in other contexts should be used only with the sender's permission. In short, treat information from e-mail as you would that obtained by conventional mail.

Discussion Groups

As well as using e-mail for one-to-one communication, you can join Internet discussion groups on medical topics of interest. Likewise, you can take part in newsgroups maintained by commercial online services. Online and printed Internet guides, as well as people knowledgeable in given fields, can direct you to such groups. The Web site Deja News at http://www.reference.com lets you search for newsgroups on given topics and also provides access to recent postings from the groups.

"There's a support group for everything online," one freelance writer observes. Monitoring the messages can yield story ideas, alert you to patients' concerns, and aid in identifying people to interview. And posting messages of your own can lead you to information and sources. If you post messages for such purposes, ethics requires that you indicate that you are seeking the material for a story. And of course, good journalistic practice demands that you verify all information.

Online resources have much to offer health writers. Keep informed about them, and use them wisely. They will help free you from constraints of time, place, the mails, and the telephone.

PART II

Preparing the Piece

Chapter 6

EVALUATING INFORMATION

While gathering information for possible use in your story, you doubtless have been starting to evaluate it. Now, as you integrate material from various sources, further evaluation is crucial. This chapter discusses ten key items to consider when deciding what information to present and in what context to present it. Some examples of applying material from this chapter are included in the annotated health stories that accompany Chapter 8.

On reading some sections of this chapter, you may feel at first that nothing you find is good enough to present. Do not despair. Remember that medicine is an evolving field and that your role as a health writer often is to convey an understanding of what is known—and isn't known—at present. You need not reject all that may be flawed in some way; indeed, if you did, you might have little to say. Rather, reject that which has serious weaknesses, make clear the limitations of other material, and remember to present information in a broad enough context for your audience to see how it fits in.

The Source

In deciding how much credence to assign, consider the information source. Knowing the source helps in determining how confident you can be that information was competently gathered and analyzed. It also can alert you to possible bias.

Consider, for example, where research was reported. Was it published in a peer-reviewed journal? Or was it presented only at a conference, which typically would have much less stringent quality control?

If research was reported in a journal, what affiliations are listed for the authors? For example, do the authors work for a university, the government, or a pharmaceutical company? Also, what institutions are listed as funding the research? Was the research supported by a government agency? by industry? by a private foundation? Do there seem to be possible conflicts of interest? For instance, is an article evaluating a medical device accompanied by a statement that the author has been a consultant to the company producing the device?

II. Preparing the Piece

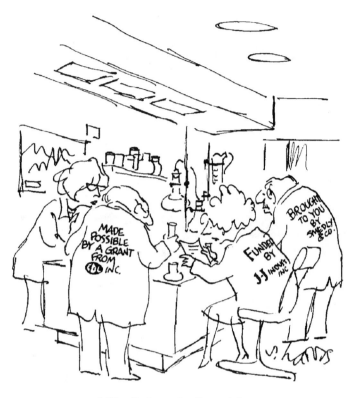

© Sidney Harris, reproduced by permission.

When researchers, health professionals, and others make pronounce-
ments, are they indeed experts on the subjects they are addressing? Or are
they speaking outside their areas of expertise? Who pays their salaries,
gives them consulting fees, or supports their research? With what causes
are they known to be affiliated?

And when information comes from an institution, what are the institution's funding sources and goals? If an institution has an ambiguous
name, what does the institution actually represent and do? For example, is
it is funded by a given industry and geared to advancing its interests? Is an
association about to launch a fundraising drive and thus trying to engender publicity?

Clearly, circumstantial evidence such as that on the nature of sources is
not always valid. Work done by researchers at top universities and published in respected journals has later turned out to be fraudulent. And in-

6. Evaluating Information

formation and ideas from well outside the mainstream have turned out to be valid and important.

Nevertheless, consider the source when deciding what stories to pursue and what information to include. And provide sufficient information on the source so that your audience also can consider it.

Consistency

Think about consistency, both within a source and from source to source. If you are looking at a research article, are the numbers in the text consistent with those listed in the tables? Do the conclusions seem consistent with the data reported? If inconsistencies appear to exist, are they serious enough to disqualify the article from consideration or to merit contacting the researcher for a possible interpretation?

If you obtained statistics on a given item—say, the number of people with a certain disease—are those from different sources similar? If not, are the statistics central enough to your story that it would be worth looking into possible reasons for the discrepancies? Or would it suffice to provide a range of estimates?

If you are writing about a given piece of research, are its findings consistent with those of other studies that have attempted to address the same question? Different findings do not necessarily mean that one study is wrong and another is right. Rather, they often reflect the fact that different studies looked at different aspects of the same question—for example, effects of a treatment in different populations. However, such discrepancies are indeed worth reflecting on and noting.

The Study Design

Inconsistencies in the findings of different studies often reflect, in part, differences in study design. Not all studies are created equal. For health writers, the advantages and limitations of various study designs are important to consider when evaluating information.

In health writing and other popular writing, anecdotes often bring dull generalities to life. But beware, beware, beware of depending only on anecdotal information. Although a patient's unfavorable experience—say, with a medication or a given type of health-care facility—can well be a starting point for research into a possible story, it is by no means grounds in itself for a story concluding that the item in question is bad. And do not conclude that a treatment is effective just because one patient's condition improved. Most conditions have their ups and downs, and improvement can be independent of any treatment. Thus, a comparison or control group receiving no treatment or an established treatment almost always is needed before one can validly conclude that a treatment is effective or an improvement. Other things being equal, the greater the number of people studied, the more credible the results of the research.

For evaluating treatments and preventive measures, the type of study generally considered to be the gold standard is the randomized double-blind controlled clinical trial. *Randomized* means that patients or subjects are randomly assigned to groups; without randomization, an investigator may, for example, tend to assign sicker patients to receive one treatment or another. *Double-blind* means that neither the investigators nor the study participants know who is receiving which treatment; this removes a source of possible bias in evaluating responses. (When use of medication is being compared with use of no medication, members of the control group receive placebos—pills that contain no active agent but look like the real thing. Of course, studies of some kinds of treatment, such as those comparing the use of medication and the use of surgery, cannot be double-blind.) *Controlled* means that a comparison or control group was included in the study. In general, randomized controlled clinical trials, especially those reported in major medical journals, are studies in which health writers can place considerable credence.

Clinical trials are not always feasible or reasonable to do. Nor are they suited to address everything worthy of study. Consider, for example, research on whether smoking affects the likelihood of developing a given disease. Scientifically, the soundest approach may be to assign people randomly to become smokers or not and then watch for development of the disease. However, even if doing so were practical, it would not be ethical. Also, sometimes factors being studied are beyond human control and thus unsuited for an experimental approach. For example, researchers may wish to determine whether a genetic trait affects the likelihood of developing a given disease in the hope of diagnosing and treating the disease early in those so predisposed. The researchers cannot give people the trait; rather, to seek their answer, they must observe people who have it.

In circumstances such as these, researchers take observational approaches rather than conducting experiments such as controlled clinical trials. Sometimes the research is *prospective,* or forward-looking, such as when it follows groups of smokers and nonsmokers over the years and compares their health condition. Other times the research is *retrospective,* or backward-looking. Such research compares groups with and without a given disease or condition in search of differences that could have predisposed those affected to develop the disease.

One difficulty in interpreting such observational studies is ascertaining whether a factor found to be associated with a condition actually contributes to causing the condition or whether it is merely linked with another factor that, in turn, is causal. If more smokers do develop a certain condition, is smoking itself responsible? Or could it be that people who choose to smoke tend toward other habits that increase the likelihood of developing the condition? If a retrospective study finds that people who have been treated for cancer are at increased risk of later developing a second cancer, is the treatment indeed responsible, or could the new cancer reflect the same factors that led to the original one? For aid in considering such questions, look at the discussion sections of journal articles reporting observational studies. Also look for related editorials in the same issue of the journal.

Some studies seek to determine how people's health condition changes with age. In general, the ideal approach is to observe the same group for many years. However, such *longitudinal* studies sometimes are impractical, and, of course, the results are slow to obtain. Therefore, researchers sometimes undertake *cross-sectional* studies, which compare people of various ages regarding aspects of interest. If, however, a cross-sectional study discloses differences, one difficulty is knowing whether the differences are indeed due to age or whether the older people always differed from the younger people, for example, because of differences in their childhood diets. Here, too, look for discussion in articles presenting the research and in accompanying editorials.

Some health research involves gathering information from patients or members of the public. Here, consider whether the study design may have limited the accuracy of responses. For example, in a retrospective study, were subjects asked about events long ago that they may not have recalled clearly? Or in an interview survey on health habits, might subjects have tended to give what they perceived to be the socially correct response? Such a questioning attitude, which traditionally marks the good reporter, certainly marks the good health writer considering study design.

For further consideration of study design, one health-writer-friendly source is the book *News and Numbers: A Guide to Reporting Statistical Claims and Controversies in Health and Other Fields* (Cohn 1994). Written by Victor

II. Preparing the Piece

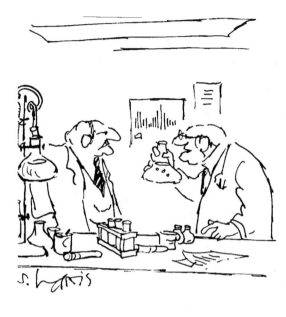

"IT MAY VERY WELL BRING ABOUT IMMORTALITY, BUT IT WILL TAKE FOREVER TO TEST IT."

Cohn, who long covered health and medicine for the *Washington Post*, this work is an excellent resource on both study design and statistics, the topic of the next section.

The Numbers

Evaluating information on health often entails interpreting numbers. As a health writer you need not be a master statistician. Rather, familiarity with the basic items below, along with a thoughtful attitude, will accomplish much of what you need.

An example where a bit more thinking might have helped: A magazine listed the numbers of deaths estimated to occur per year in various cities as a result of tiny particles polluting the air. Those cities with the most such deaths, the author implied, were those with the deadliest air. But those with the most such deaths tended to be merely the largest cities. Before making comparisons, the writer should have divided each number by the city's population and thus come up with rates. Only then could the cities be compared meaningfully.

Little more than alertness and common sense can suffice for avoiding pitfalls such as that above, but considering numbers is difficult at times. When you find yourself beyond your depth, written resources include basic, everyday-oriented statistics books such as *Seeing Through Statistics* (Utts 1996), as well as the above-mentioned *News and Numbers* (Cohn 1994). Human sources—such as study authors and public health officials—can, and often should, be consulted for aid in interpreting the statistics they provided.

Statisticians uninvolved in the work or situation being reported also can be valuable resources. "Make friends with someone in your local statistics department," advises a health writer who is himself a researcher. Public information staff at universities can help you find statisticians available to consult.

When in doubt, do ask a statistics expert for professional guidance. "Always trust your instinct if something doesn't sit right," another experienced health writer states. "Check, check, check."

Health-Related Rates

Incidence. Prevalence. Morbidity. Mortality. Even if only an aspiring health writer, you probably have heard these terms. And quite likely have heard them misused.

The *incidence rate* indicates how common the occurrence of new cases of a given disease or condition was in a given population over a given period. Say, for example, that you live in a city of 100,000. And say that last year 530 people in your city developed the mythical disease healthwriters' syndrome. You could then state that the incidence rate last year was 530 per 100,000 (or 5.3 per 1,000). And you could compare the incidence rate last year with that in previous years to see whether the tendency to develop the disease was changing. You could also compare the incidence rate with those in other cities to determine whether people in your city appeared more or less prone to the disease.

However, you should best take care in interpreting the incidence rates of healthwriters' disease. Do the rates include all new cases of the disease, or only those for which treatment was sought from a doctor? Were rates ascertained similarly over time—or, for example, did increased coverage in the media last year lead more people to seek medical attention for their healthwriters' disease? Were cases of healthwriters' disease sometimes concealed because it is considered a shameful condition? In preparing stories that rely heavily on statistics such as incidence rates, answers to such questions can be well worth obtaining.

Incidence rates do not say what proportion of people in a population have a given condition at a given time, but *prevalence rates* do. If healthwriters' disease is a fleeting affliction, such as a cold, perhaps only 10 people in your city have the disease today; thus, the prevalence rate would be 10 per 100,000. But if healthwriters' disease is a chronic nonfatal condition developing in early life, the prevalence rate would much exceed the incidence rate.

Morbidity means disease. Thus, both incidence rates and prevalence rates are *morbidity rates*. (Sometimes, though, "morbidity rate" is used to mean "incidence rate"; if in doubt what is meant, be sure to ask.) In contrast, *mortality* means death, and *mortality rates* are death rates. You can write about the total death rate in a population over a given period. You can also write about the death rate attributable to a given disease; for example, if 300 people died of disease X last year in your city of 100,000, the death rate from disease X last year would be 300 per 100,000 (or 3 per 1,000). You can also write about case fatality rates—that is, the proportion of cases of a given disease that result in death. If on average 8 of every 10 people with disease X die of it, the case fatality rate is 80 percent.

When comparing rates, make sure the rates used are valid for the comparison being drawn. Let's say you find the incidence of heart attacks in your city to be much lower than that in a neighboring city. Can you surmise that people in your city probably have lifestyles that help prevent heart attacks? What if your city is a university town and the other city is a retirement community? Clearly, some adjustment for age is needed, and indeed *age-adjusted rates* exist. When logic tells you that the rates you have are not sufficient for the comparisons you wish to make, call on an expert for help.

Response Rates

For the health writer, another important number to consider is the *rate of response* to surveys. If a health-related survey was sent to the people in your community and only 10 percent of the recipients responded, might those 10 percent have differed from your community's overall population?

Quite likely. Should you doubt that the findings accurately reflect the situation in your community? Yes indeed.

In short, whether a survey is of an entire population or of a sample thereof, look carefully at the response rate. If the rate was low, be cautious in what—if anything—you conclude.

Averages and Ranges

Some of the most basic statistics are *averages*. Simple as they may seem, they can be misused or at least misleading.

Often, "average" is construed only to mean *mean*—that is, the arithmetic average obtained by adding up all the values and dividing by the number of values. If values are evenly distributed around a center point, the mean can provide a good indication of what is typical. Let's say, however, that the distribution is skewed. What if the typical case of our mythical disease healthwriters' syndrome costs $50 to treat—but in one case in 1,000, life-threatening complications develop, requiring extensive hospital treatment at a cost of $100,000? The mean cost of treating the syndrome is then about $150. This mean value can aid in assigning appropriate resources, but it does not show what is typical. In cases of such skewed distributions, another type of average, the *median*—or middle value, when all the values are listed from lowest to highest—can provide a truer indication of the norm. So, sometimes, can the *mode*—the most common value. And describing the distribution, as was done above, is sometimes the best approach of all.

Also, values can be narrowly or widely distributed around a given mean or median. And different distributions—whether of survival times, costs, ages, or other items pertinent to health—can have different implications. Thus consider obtaining and providing information on distributions.

In short, when evaluating information, try to make sure that the statistics used to describe a situation give a sufficiently complete and accurate picture. If in doubt, seek fuller information.

Percent Change

One figure commonly presented in health writing—and, it seems, commonly computed wrong—is *percent change*. The key: In computing percent change, always use the initial value as the baseline, not the later value.

Imagine that last year 100 people in your community received a given treatment. What if 120 people received the treatment this year? Then the number of people receiving the treatment increased by 20 percent. Or what if 80 people received the treatment this year? Then the number decreased by 20 percent. In either case, the change was 20 out of the initial 100—or 20 percent. The change was not, in the latter case, 20 out of 80, or 25 percent, because 80 was the later value, not the initial one.

Relative Risk

One of the statistics most commonly encountered by health writers is *relative risk,* sometimes called risk ratio. Simply put, relative risk indicates by what mathematical factor, if at all, an item such as an exposure or habit appears to affect the likelihood of developing a given condition. For example, if exposure to chemical X is associated with double the usual likelihood of developing condition Y, then the relative risk is 2.0. If the exposure is associated with half the usual likelihood, the relative risk is one-half, or 0.5. And if the likelihood is unchanged, the relative risk is 1.0.

Although relative risk helps show how strongly a factor seems to affect the likelihood of developing a given condition, it presents only part of the picture. Information also is needed on the absolute magnitude of the risk. Let's say that with regard to a given type of cancer, exposure to chemical Z is associated with a relative risk of 10. This relative risk is high. However, if the type of cancer is normally very rare—say, affecting only one person in one million—even relatively widespread exposure will result in few extra cases. And say that with regard to another type of cancer, exposure to chemical Z is associated with a relative risk of 2. Clearly, this relative risk is much lower. But if the cancer is a much more common type—say, affecting one person in one hundred—even this relative risk will result in many extra cases.

In short, when evaluating information, do not let relative risk suffice (unless the value is one). Rather, obtain information on absolute risk as well.

Statistical Significance

Statistical significance. Sounds important. And indeed it is an important concept to grasp. However, it indicates only how likely it is that findings reflect more than a chance association. It in no way indicates how much practical importance the findings have.

In journal articles and conference talks, statistical significance often is presented in terms of *P values,* or probability values. Put simply, the P value is the probability (expressed as a decimal) that an effect at least as large as that observed could have occurred by chance if in fact there had been no real effect. Thus, the smaller the P value, the greater the certainty that the observed difference—for example, in the effectiveness of two drugs—reflected a real difference, not merely reflect chance variation. Often, to accept results as sufficiently credible, researchers require P values to be less than 0.05—meaning that chances are lower than 1 in 20 that the observed effect was just an artefact of chance. If, for example, the P value is 0.001 (one in a thousand), considerably more certainty can be attached to the results.

Another way that biomedical papers and talks sometimes present statistical significance is in terms of *confidence intervals*, which are akin to the "margins of error" sometimes reported for surveys such as political polls. Simply put, a confidence interval is the range within which one can be 95 percent sure that the actual value lies. For instance, say that on the basis of findings of a study, a relative risk is estimated to be 1.9. A 95 percent confidence interval then calculated to be 1.3 to 2.8 means that chances are 95 percent that the actual relative risk falls within that range. The wider the confidence interval, the less precise the estimate. For relative risk, reporting a confidence interval that overlaps 1.0—say, one that ranges from 0.5 to 4.5—is another way of saying that findings are not statistically significant.

Being statistically significant does not necessarily mean that something is of practical importance. Consider, for example, a study that finds a small but statistically significant difference in how long two drugs require to take effect. Statistical significance means that one can be reasonably confident that the speeds do differ along the lines described. However, it does not say whether the findings are of clinical importance. If the disease being treated is life-threatening and every second counts, the difference could be vital indeed. But if the ailment is minor, the difference may be of no real consequence, and other differences between the two drugs—such as cost or side effects—may be of overriding importance.

Power

Lack of statistical significance does not mean that an effect does not exist. It means only that from a given study one cannot conclude with reasonable confidence that an effect indeed exists.

Put another way, absence of proof is not proof of absence. A study may have been incapable of detecting an effect even if one existed. Or put more technically, the study may have lacked what is known as statistical power. Just as a powerful microscope is needed to see small microorganisms, a statistically powerful study is needed to validly discern small differences between the test groups.

Little power is needed to test a possible cure for a normally fatal disorder such as rabies. If the treatment actually is a cure, testing it on just a few patients will show its value. In contrast, a powerful study involving many patients would be needed to test whether a drug improves the survival rate of patients with a condition that rarely is fatal.

When reading journal articles reporting that findings were not statistically significant, look in the discussion section for a discussion of statistical power. If you do not find such discussion, ask the investigator about the power of the study to detect the difference sought.

Statistical power increases and confidence intervals narrow as the size of the study population grows. Thus, all other things being equal, large studies tend to be more credible than small ones. But beware of a common fallacy: Sometimes when a small study shows a difference that fails to reach statistical significance, people say that had the study been larger, a statistically significant difference would have been found. However, all they can validly say is that had the study been larger, it would have been more capable of finding convincing evidence of an effect, if indeed such an effect existed.

Clusters

Over a short period, several cases of an uncommon disease are detected in a small community. Some people in the community suspect that something in the environment is responsible. How would you, as a health writer, proceed?

The way to proceed is with caution. The rates might not actually exceed those normally occurring. Or the *cluster* of cases might not be larger than those expected to occur from time to time by chance. To find whether the numbers are worthy of suspicion, consult experts on public health.

Interpretations

Findings are just that. Findings. They can be interpreted in various ways. When you receive information, consider the interpretations provided. Think whether they make sense to you. See whether you or others can think of plausible alternatives.

In particular, beware of assuming that *correlation* necessarily means *causality*, or that the causality necessarily runs in a given direction. Consider, for instance, a study finding that older people who continue to be employed are healthier, on average, than those who have retired. Some might conclude that continuing to work helps keep one healthy. But could the findings have reflected, at least in part, the fact that only people who are healthy enough can continue to work?

When evaluating information, try to come up with alternative interpretations yourself. Look for them in discussion sections of journal articles and ask researchers and other experts about them. If they appear worthy of further consideration, share them with your audience.

Applicability

Although the conclusions of a study might be well grounded, they might not necessarily apply to the audience your health writing serves. The conclusions may have been drawn from a study only of people with a given disease. Or the study may have been done in a specialized population such as nuns or nurses or doctors. Or the researchers may have studied only men, only young people, or only people of a given race. Indeed, the researchers may not have studied people at all but rather animals—or molecules. Thus, questions can—and should—exist about whether the findings apply to populations for whom you are writing.

As a health writer evaluating information, you should notice these possible limitations to applicability and note them in your writing. Find out whether studies in various groups or experimental systems have yielded similar findings, thus strengthening the likelihood that the conclusions can validly be *generalized*. Check the discussion sections of journal articles for discussions of the generalizability of the findings and discuss the matter with authors and other experts. Beware of generalizing too much from information you encounter.

Alternatives

Often a given source, such as a journal article, deals with only a single approach or a limited range of approaches. Considering alternatives can result in sounder, more useful health writing.

Say that a journal article reports a study comparing two surgical operations. The condition being treated is common, and you decide to write about the findings. But are these operations the only approaches? What about other operations? How about treatment with medication? How about lifestyle measures? Does the condition demand treatment, or can one get along without it?

Answering such questions helps distinguish the thoughtful, analytical health writer from the mere scribe or parrot.

Uniqueness

Too often, it seems, we assume that that which is new is unique. For the health writer, checking whether this assumption holds is part of evaluating information. Has a new drug been approved for release? Check whether the drug is truly novel or merely a variant of an existing drug. Has a research article of possible interest been published? Check whether the work is a new departure or rather part of a body of related research by one

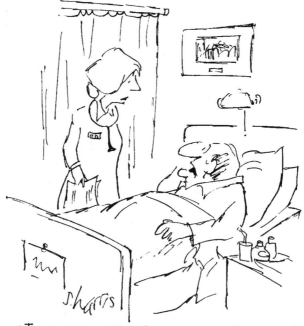

"I STOPPED TAKING THE MEDICINE BECAUSE I PREFER THE ORIGINAL DISEASE TO THE SIDE EFFECTS."

© Sidney Harris, reproduced by permission.

or more groups. Or is a local hospital opening a new kind of clinic or acquiring equipment of a new type? Check whether other facilities offer similar services or plan to do so. Such checking can help provide important context.

The Big Picture

Alternatives and uniqueness are parts of the big picture. Depending on the topic, other parts can include such items as the history of a situation, implications for the future, social and ethical and legal aspects, and economics. Considering such items often entails one of the hardest parts of evaluating information: determining what information is initially missing and readily gathered. But conceptualizing the big picture—and understanding and presenting it—can be well worth the effort.

The Costs

Costs have become such an important part of the big picture regarding health that they merit separate mention. No longer does it suffice—if it ever did—to say that a medical technology is an advance. Rather, in a world of limited resources, the costs of technologies require consideration. So, too, the monetary and human costs of much else regarding health.

Such consideration will cost you some time and effort, as will other aspects of evaluating information for writing about health. With experience, however, your efficiency will increase. And, from the beginning, the payoff will be a sounder basis for your piece.

Chapter 7

ΗΕΑLΤΗ-WRITING TECHNIQUE

Good health writing is at heart good writing. It relies on the same approaches and techniques. However, some items are particularly important in health writing, which can pose special challenges.

This chapter identifies approaches and techniques especially pertinent to health writing and discusses their use. As well as dealing with crafting a piece of health writing, it looks at gearing the piece to the audience and checking it for accuracy. In keeping with its own advice, the chapter includes examples. Readers with limited background in writing are encouraged to read one or more general guides to effective writing. One highly readable, widely available such guide is *On Writing Well* (Zinsser 1994). Also recommended, though dated in some respects, is *The Elements of Style* (Strunk and White 1979).

Assessing the Audience

A few years ago, when the hazards of excessive sun exposure were becoming increasingly apparent, a variety of magazines ran articles on protection from the sun. Articles in *Redbook, Working Woman, Esquire, Parents, Business Week,* and *Outdoor Life* contained similar basic information. Each, however, had a different emphasis, in keeping with the magazine's focus and audience. The *Parents* piece focused on protecting babies from the sun, the *Esquire* article showcased the views of leading male skiers, and the *Working Woman* story included information on the sunscreen industry.

Before crafting a piece of health writing, assess the audience. Consider its age, its education, its knowledge level, its interests. Consider whether the piece should have a local emphasis. Look carefully at other articles in the same publication, or listen carefully to other stories on the same broadcast program. Pay particular attention to the vocabulary level, lest you, having reviewed materials such as journal articles, tend to lapse into technical jargon. Check with the editor, who is likely to be well attuned to the audience being served.

Consider checking as well with members of the potential audience, or with people of similar background and interests. One experienced writing teacher suggests the following approach: Mention to people that you plan to do a story on a given topic, then listen to their reactions. Do people say "oh yuck" or "oh boy"? Are they knowledgeable about the topic? Do they voice myths and misconceptions? Are there aspects they wonder about? Finding out can aid in deciding on both content and approach.

Beginning Effectively

Get off to a good beginning, and quite likely the rest of your piece will work well. Do not despair, though, if the beginning is slow in coming. Devising a good beginning entails much hard thinking—such as clarifying to yourself the central point of the piece and deciding on an appropriate structure. Once you have a good beginning in place, usually the rest goes much faster.

A good beginning both engages the audience and makes clear what the piece is about. In a news story, the beginning, or lead, typically accomplishes these goals quickly. Consider these leads from newspaper articles:

> Americans finally can prevent that itchy and sometimes dangerous rite of childhood: The government approved the nation's first chickenpox vaccine Friday. (Neergaard 1995)

> Alzheimer's disease may stalk its victims early in life, decades before it destroys the mind, a study of nuns who are donating their brains to science suggests. (Coleman 1996a)

> Most of the 11 million Americans with heart disease can relax and enjoy sex if they want—it's highly unlikely to trigger a heart attack, a study found. (Coleman 1996b)

Each of these leads gets to the main point quickly. And because the topics are newsworthy, the subject matter itself helps make each lead engaging.

Feature stories often begin more slowly. Here is a lead from a newspaper piece on the high demand to hire family practitioners and other primary care physicians:

> One classified ad rhapsodizes about "lake homes, low cost of living, nonexistent crime and great schools." Others sing of incredible scenery, amazing fishing, astounding golf courses.

7. Technique

Selling time-share condos, perhaps? Franchise opportunities?
No, these ads in the back pages of medical journals are a window on an even hotter market: the competition for family doctors. (Haney 1994)

This lead uses vivid images and lively wording, as well as suspense and surprise, to entice the reader. But it also makes clear what the topic of the story will be. Implicitly it tells the reader: Even if physician employment didn't interest you much before, read on; this article will be interesting.

Finally, consider a longer lead that draws on various techniques useful in health writing:

> In nearly every room of Kevin Leitzell's house on a shady street in suburban Philadelphia sits a footstool. Dangling from the light switches are long plastic rods, and the lock on the back door measures inches lower than on most doors. Parked in the driveway is Kevin's '94 Ford Escort, and if you peek through the window you'll see extensions on the pedals that elevate the surfaces more than a foot.
>
> At 17, Kevin is a junior at Haverford Township Senior High and stands an even 4 feet tall. He is an achondroplastic dwarf who uses footstools, pedal extensions and the like to compensate for his short stature. He's also sports editor of the school paper, manager of both the soccer and baseball teams, and working on getting a date for the prom. There is nothing in the demeanor of this young man, who hopes for a career in radio broadcasting or sports reporting, to indicate that he will allow his short limbs or any of the host of other physical problems that can accompany achondroplasia to limit his ambitions.
>
> On this day, Kevin greets a visitor with a friendly smile. "My attitude toward the world," he explains, in answer to a question about everyday difficulties, "is like it or not, here I come!"
>
> It's an outlook that has been nourished and supported by the Johns Hopkins Center for Medical Genetics ... (Henderson and Centofanti 1995)

This lead from an article in the magazine *Hopkins Medical News* engages readers in various ways. Like the previous lead, it contains suspense. It also includes considerable human interest. As writers are often advised to do, the authors show rather than tell: Readers see that people like Kevin can have largely normal lives but must make some adjustments. Also fulfilling its second function, this lead indicates what the article will be about—people with dwarfism and the medical services for them at Johns Hopkins. It also introduces more specific themes of the piece, such as the medical problems to which people with dwarfism are prone.

As you read health writing, look for engaging, informative leads. And strive to write such leads yourself.

II. Preparing the Piece

Explaining Well

Much health writing involves explanation. Skillful health writers have long used various techniques to make their explanations effective. In addition, research (Rowan 1990) supports using some less widely known measures.

Explaining Terms and Concepts

Health writers often must explain what unfamiliar terms mean. Presenting the concept before the new term can ease understanding and help keep from intimidating readers. An example of this technique: In an article on osteoporosis (Travis 1995), the author writes of "bone-forming cells called osteoblasts" and "their destructive kin, the bone-destroying osteoclasts."

Although you may define a term, readers may not remember its meaning. Thus, if you reuse it after a while, consider providing a brief reminder. For example, early in a piece about a bone-marrow disease (Weaver 1994), the marrow is noted to contain "a delicate network of fibers known as reticulin." Later, when the term "reticulin" is used again, it is immediately followed by the reminder phrase "the fibers in the marrow."

Also, examples can help clarify terms or concepts. For instance, in his popular piece "Germs," physician-essayist Lewis Thomas states,

> Most bacteria are totally preoccupied with browsing, altering the configurations of organic molecules so that they become usable for the energy needs of other forms of life. They are, by and large, indispensable to each other, living in interdependent communities in the soil or sea. Some have become symbionts in more specialized, local relations, living as working parts in the tissues of higher organisms.

Hmmm. Rather abstract and hard to visualize. But soon Thomas adds some examples:

> The root nodules of legumes would have neither form nor function without the masses of rhizobial bacteria swarming into root hairs, incorporating themselves with such intimacy that only an electron microscope can detect which membranes are bacterial and which plant. Insects have colonies of bacteria, the mycetocytes, living in them like little glands, doing heaven knows what but being essential. The microfloras of animal intestinal tracts are part of the nutri-

tional system. And then, of course, there are the mitochondria and chloroplasts, permanent residents in everything. (Thomas 1974)

Aah, much clearer. Also more vivid and memorable.

Showing How Things Work

Health writing often entails explaining how things work. Consider this explanation of how the medication L-dopa helps control the neurologic disorder Parkinson's disease:

> In the brain this compound [L-dopa] is transformed into dopamine, a vital chemical that is lacking in Parkinson's patients. Normally dopamine is produced by a specific set of nerve cells called the substantia nigra, tucked away at the base of the brain. The dopamine acts as a messenger, or neurotransmitter, and allows the substantia nigra to control one of the major motor areas in the brain, the striatum. But if there is no dopamine to act on the receptors of the striatal neurons, the patient develops Parkinson's disease. The striatum itself, however, remains normal in Parkinson's patients. So if the lost messenger can be replaced, the patients improve. And that's the role of L-dopa. (Klawans 1991)

This explanation appeared in the science magazine *Discover* and thus may be more technical than those normally appearing in media such as newspapers. Nevertheless, it is easy to follow for a number of reasons. First, the author describes the process in stepwise fashion. Also, he uses transitional words—such as "this," "but," and "so"—to show the relationships of ideas. Perhaps less obviously, he also ties ideas together by repeating the same key words in successive sentences; the term "dopamine" appears in each of the first four sentences, and words such as "patient(s)" and "messenger" also are repeated in the paragraph. (In such explanations, unlike in some more literary writing, promoting clarity through use of consistent wording takes priority over using a varied vocabulary.) Finally, in keeping with an earlier suggestion, concepts tend to be presented before the technical terms for them. The author writes of "a specific set of nerve cells called the substantia nigra" and "a messenger, or neurotransmitter."

Analogies, too, can aid in showing how things function. Consider the following use of analogy to explain how fever arises:

> A part of our brain called the hypothalamus functions much like a thermostat. Normally it is set for 98.6 degrees. If body temperature drops below that,

you shiver to generate heat, divert blood from the periphery of your body to vital organs, and pile on the blankets. Temperatures above 98.6 cause you to sweat and breathe faster to dissipate heat. What IL-1 [interleukin-1, a body chemical involved in producing fever] does is cause the set point to shift upward. In other words, you begin to feel cold at 98.6, and various warming responses kick in and a new equilibrium is reached at a higher temperature. You are now running a fever. (Sapolsky 1990)

Here, comparison of the body's temperature-control system to a familiar device, the thermostat, makes the mechanism of fever easier to understand. Note that as well as presenting an analogy, this passage uses other, previously mentioned techniques to make the explanation clear. Among them are repetition (the recurring 98.6's) and use of transitional words and phrases ("in other words" and "now").

Often researchers accustomed to explaining their work to those outside their fields present analogies during interviews. Thus, when talking with experts, be alert for analogies that can clarify your explanations. If the analogies are apt but not worded suitably for your audience, recast them in your own words but credit your source; you might say that "Dr. ___ compares ___ to ___" and then present the comparison in your own terms. When your sources' words work well as is, you can quote them directly—thus providing both the clarity and liveliness of a good analogy and the engagingness of a good quote.

An example of quoting an analogy comes from a passage explaining how genes such as oncogenes influence development of cancer. Here the researcher is quoted as follows:

The automobile is a good analogy of what happens. The oncogenes are in normal cells but have mutated and gone awry, acquiring the potential to trigger abnormal cell division. The oncogenes act as accelerators for cell growth. It is like having the car in top gear with the accelerator stuck to the floor. But just like the driver of a car can reverse a floored accelerator by stepping on the brakes, so can other genes brake the oncogenes.

The cell's brakes are called tumor-suppressor genes ... (Breo 1994)

Be alert for such analogies as you interview.

Graphics such as diagrams and flow charts also can aid considerably in showing how things work. Including them may especially aid those audience members who are more attuned to pictures than to words. Even if you are mainly a "word person," look for suitable types of graphics during your information search and think how your material might be presented visually; perhaps develop some sketches. Then share this material with the art staff if you write for a site that has one. Whether developing graphics yourself, choosing from those available, or working with others who prepare them, strive for simple graphics that present key elements without clutter that can distract. Your efforts can produce an explanation that is clearer and more appealing than otherwise and reaches a broader audience.

Countering Misconceptions

Not surprisingly, given the importance of health to people's lives but the many gaps that have existed in medical understanding, there are many misconceptions relating to health. Often the health writer's task of explaining includes countering these misconceptions, which often seem plausible but can lead to behaviors (or lack thereof) detrimental to health.

Drawing on research in science education, communication scholar Katherine E. Rowan (1990) has suggested a strategy for countering such misconceptions and providing more scientifically accepted explanations in their place. Rowan recommends beginning by stating people's common, often intuitive view and acknowledging its apparent plausibility. Only then, she advises, should one demonstrate the inadequacy of this view, state what is more scientifically founded, and show its greater adequacy.

As an example of such a "transformative explanation," Rowan offers the following passage written by a student:

> New parents sometimes object to constant use of child-restraint seats [in automobiles], thinking that their newborns must be just as safe in adult laps and firmly wrapped arms as they would be in restraint seats. The idea seems reasonable at first since babies weigh so little.
>
> But what it fails to account for is the car's speed. In a collision at 30 mph both parent and child continue to travel at 30 mph after impact. A mother could no more hold on to her child in the car than she could if she were falling out of a three-story building—on top of the child! The force of the impact in both cases would be essentially the same.

By assessing—and respecting—the audience, health writers can develop such explanations well geared to counter misconceptions.

Providing Orientation

When encountering explanations or other materials that are technical or otherwise unfamiliar, audience members can easily become lost. You can help orient them by indicating the direction in which your piece is heading.

One useful orientation device shown in some of the passages above is the use of transitional words and phrases (some further examples: "also," "therefore," "next," "in contrast," "for instance," "finally"). Another such device is the use of headings to let readers know what is coming and help them find material again. And a third device is the presentation of overviews before details—say, telling readers that a process has three steps before presenting the steps, or presenting the essence of an analogy before describing the details.

Health writers often intuitively provide orientation through such devices. Nevertheless, some explicit attention can be in order. If you sense that a passage may be confusing, check whether you seem to be providing sufficient orientation.

Providing Points of Entry

Readers are attracted to a piece in different ways. Some are drawn by the headline or title or by headings within the piece. Others are captured by the lead or by quotations drawn from the story and set in larger type. Still others are enticed by a photograph or drawing. And some are drawn in by other elements, such as brief related articles, or "sidebars," accompanying the main piece.

Health writing offers many chances to provide such "points of entry." Given the widespread interest in health, titles and headlines that attract readers can be readily crafted. And given the human and scientific elements in health care and medical research, there are many opportunities for photographs and other graphics. Depending on the type of piece, opportunities also may exist for sidebars—sets of tips, brief profiles of researchers or patients, deeper explanations for readers wanting further detail, or lists of sources of further information or help.

Whether you write or edit pieces on health, keep in mind opportunities for such points of entry. Doing so can help you engage your readers—and thus get your message across.

Including Human Interest

A strong way to engage the audience is through human interest. Fortunately, opportunity for human interest abounds in writing about health.

7. Technique

There are patients, health professionals, researchers, and other players. And of course various health topics relate to many of us as individuals and to others important in our lives.

Still or moving photographs of people involved add human interest; and in depicting signs of a disease, they can be worth at least a good fraction of the oft-mentioned 1,000 words. Anecdotes—say, of how a health condition affected a given patient's life—also add human interest, as well as serving as examples to help convey concepts. One caution, though: Do not abuse the human element. Although depictions of the bizarre and extreme, or pitiful tales of patients' woes, may initially draw audience members to a piece, they are the stuff of supermarket tabloids, not of good health writing.

Quotations from patients, scientists, and others also can add human interest and enliven a piece. However, they should be used sparingly, lest they lose their impact. Typically, they should not be used to convey routine information such as definitions or statistics; you generally can present such information most clearly and concisely, as well as most suitably for your audience, yourself.

Three items for which quotations can indeed be useful in health writing are adding color through speakers' lively wording, conveying experts' views, and showing how people feel. Two examples of quotes providing liveliness and authority come from an article on keeping one's kitchen clean in order to prevent foodborne disease:

> "Bacteria are all in business for themselves, and the business is making more bacteria," says George Chang, a professor of food microbiology at the University of California at Berkeley. "We're inviting the bad ones to make us sick when we don't clean properly."

and

> How to beat germs? "The biggest word in kitchen cleaning is 'now,'" says Don Aslett, author of 25 books on cleaning. (Janis 1996)

Another example of a quote providing authority comes from an article on identification of a protein playing a key role in entry of the AIDS virus into human cells:

> "There's no controversy about this. It's already been reproduced in several labs. There's no question it's correct and it's a highly significant piece of work,"

says John Moore of the Aaron Diamond AIDS Research Center in New York City. (Travis 1996)

Here are two examples of using quotations to show feelings. One is from an individual describing her first migraine headache: "It was like someone stabbing my head with an ice pick. ... It was terrifying." (Sachs 1996) And the other is from a person with arthritis: "I was frustrated. ... Arthritis made my fingers, knees and ankles so stiff that it was difficult to move them. It became harder to do the things I liked most, especially biking." (Christiano 1995)

Quotations, like photographs and anecdotes, can provide human interest and otherwise enhance health writing. Aspiring health writers inexperienced in their use can obtain further guidance from basic journalism books widely available in libraries and general and college bookstores.

Presenting Numbers and Sizes Effectively

Health writing often entails presenting numbers and sizes. One suggestion regarding numbers is to avoid presenting many such pieces of hard-to-process information at once. Rather than doing so, intersperse supporting material such as examples and quotations.

In describing sizes, comparison to familiar objects often helps. This example is from an article on asthma: A basic inhaler used to administer medication is described as "barely larger than a lipstick," whereas a more powerful device known as a nebulizer is "about twice the size of your average lunchbox." (Waldron 1993)

In short, in presenting numbers and sizes, as in presenting other technical information, try to pace yourself, and try to link the unfamiliar with the familiar. The result will be more effective health writing.

Ending Strongly

Just as the beginning of a piece can merit particular effort, so can the end. Granted, this is not always so. For example, news articles on health, like those on other topics, do not typically have formal endings; rather, they dwindle into increasing fine detail, thus allowing material to be cut from the end if space is limited. (For more on the structure of news stories, see Chapter 8.)

Feature articles on health, however, often do—and should—have endings providing closure. This example is from the article noted earlier on dwarfism and its management at Johns Hopkins:

> Young people like Eboni White and Kevin Leitzell personify a feeling of pride and self-worth common among today's generation of little people. [Note: "Little people" is a term that members of this population themselves use, not condescending wording by the article's authors.] They have had their way paved by increasing activism and antidiscrimination efforts by the Little People of America, by blunt-speaking role models like Dee Miller ("whatever you do," Miller says, sensing that a new acquaintance is not sure how to treat her, "don't pat me on the head") and, not least, by medical advances for which Johns Hopkins has been at the forefront. Step by step, those advances are allowing short-statured men and women to live longer, healthier, and more productive lives than ever before. (Henderson and Centofanti 1995)

This ending ties together various themes and people in the piece and leaves the take-home message resounding in readers' heads. If you write feature articles on health, consider striving for such a conclusion.

Providing Access to Further Information

One function of much health writing is to serve as a gateway for seeking further information. Consider whether this function is among those of your piece. If so, identify sources to mention, and present them in a way easy to find and consult.

During the research for your piece, quite likely you encountered information sources to consider mentioning to your audience. Possibilities often include government agencies such as components of the National Institutes of Health, local or national offices of health-related organizations such as the American Heart Association or American Cancer Society, and written materials. If appropriate, also mention resources such as clinics or courses. Take care, however, not to list one such resource in your vicinity while ignoring another.

"If you want to give the address or phone number of a small organization or facility in a story to be widely distributed, consider asking their permission or at least alerting them that they may soon be flooded with requests," a health writer in New Jersey advises. "I've gotten into trouble for not doing this!"

II.   Preparing the Piece

If toll-free numbers are available, provide them. Ditto for addresses of relevant sites on the World Wide Web. Given the varied quality of material on the Web, however, take care in recommending sites. If in doubt, mention only those that are associated with organizations known to be reputable.

Depending on your medium and format, you can present the sources in various ways for easy accessibility. Often, sources of further information are listed at the end of a feature article or broadcast segment. A resource list also can work well as a sidebar alongside the main article.

Finally, be sure to check the listings for accuracy and currency. Clearly, if they are incorrect or out-of-date they will frustrate rather than help.

Checking for Accuracy

Not only resource lists but also other content should be checked for accuracy. Check that you have the details right, and also make sure that you have accurately conveyed the big picture. In doing so, draw on your notes, and check reference sources. Do not hesitate to ask experts if you are unsure. Also consider having them review parts or all of your piece for technical accuracy.

In some instances, incorrect details can be harmful to readers' health. In others, they at least undermine the writer's credibility—and perhaps the writer's prospects for further health-writing assignments. Consider the following errors: One newspaper article referred to "this month's issue of the *Journal of the American Medical Association*" when this journal is published four times a month. Another placed the Mayo Clinic in Rochester, New York, rather than Rochester, Minnesota. In a single sentence, another spoke of a patient's facial ticks (should be "tics") and irritated bowel syndrome (should be "irritable bowel syndrome"). A health-related posting on the World Wide Web repeatedly said "nitrous oxide" when "nitric oxide" was meant. And the headline of a news release misspelled "laparoscopy" as "laporoscopy." Oops. Oops. Oops. By checking details you can avoid such problems.

But checking for accuracy goes beyond making sure that the details are correct. Also back away from the details and make sure that the big picture is right. If you have written about a new development, make sure you have provided sufficient context to correctly show its significance. If you have discussed an area of health where controversy exists, make sure that both

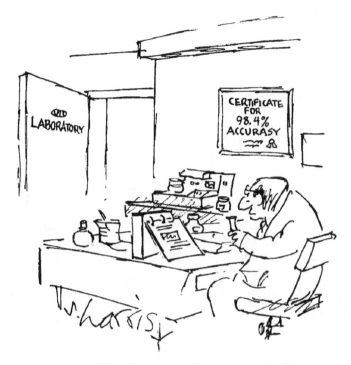

© Sidney Harris, reproduced by permission.

sides are fairly represented. It is also very important to indicate where the bulk of expert opinion lies. Whatever the nature of your article, make sure to indicate where important uncertainties exist.

If questions arise as you check your work, do not hesitate to contact sources consulted while gathering information. Technologies such as electronic mail and fax machines greatly facilitate doing so. Most sources would rather spend the time helping you check a fact than have an inaccuracy appear. Indeed, such evidence of your attention to detail may increase their willingness to work with you in the future.

Journalists traditionally have been wary about showing their drafts or parts thereof to sources for review. But views seem to be shifting (Shepard 1996). And such review has long been accepted in technical areas, including health. Passages of concern often can readily be checked by telephone, e-mail, or fax. When seeking feedback on items such as balance, a draft of an entire piece may be shown to an expert in the field. Make clear, however, that you are only seeking technically expert feedback, not ceding to others' control over your work. You remain the health writer, and the writing remains your domain.

Checking with the Audience

This chapter began with the audience. And so shall it end. Once you have drafted your piece, consider showing it to others, especially members of the intended audience or people much like them. What do people find interesting about the piece? What other information would they like to have seen? What, if anything, do they find unclear or misinterpret?

"You have to understand what people think a word means," says Ruth SoRelle, medical writer for the *Houston Chronicle*. After SoRelle wrote that genital herpes was "incurable," a man called and asked her how much longer he had to live. On talking with him, SoRelle realized that the man had confused "incurable" and "terminal." Finding out how typical readers interpret a draft can aid in revising your work to avoid such confusion.

Typically, such feedback has been obtained by showing people a draft and then asking for comments. Another approach is to obtain running comments from people while they read your draft; readers can either provide the comments directly or dictate them into a tape recorder. Yet an-

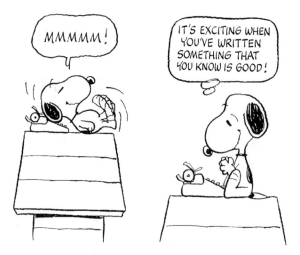

Peanuts © United Features Syndicate. Reprinted by permission.

other approach is to have a group of people read your draft and discuss it.

Serving as a representative of your audience, your editor can also provide helpful feedback. And with growing experience as a health writer, you will likely develop an "internal editor" that helps you anticipate your audience's interests and needs and check whether you have fulfilled them. If you have followed advice in this chapter, quite likely the word from readers, editors, and yourself is that you have done your job well.

Chapter 8

GENRES OF HEALTH WRITING

Health writing comes in many genres: news reports, investigative pieces, feature stories, and more. While following the conventions of these various genres, health writing also presents special challenges and concerns within them.

This chapter addresses some of the main genres in which health writers work. Examples, along with comments, underline points in the chapter and elsewhere in the book. There is also direction to sources of further guidance.

Prospective health writers without a journalism background may find it useful not only to read this chapter but also to consult basic textbooks in areas such as news writing and magazine or feature writing. And all readers are encouraged to look analytically at examples of health writing that they encounter. For whatever the genre, health writing benefits from following good models and learning to avoid errors observed in bad ones.

News Stories and News Releases

New findings. New products. New services or techniques. New personnel. Whether for the public media or in institutional settings, much health writing consists of reporting news. Whether you write a news story for the public or a news release for journalists, awareness of a few basic conventions and guidelines can aid in following an appropriate format and including appropriate information.

Both news stories and news releases typically follow what is called "inverted pyramid format." As the name implies, in this format the big stuff is up top. Thus, the opening, or lead, summarizes the news to be presented; it may also note its significance if that would be unclear. Readers then can decide whether to look at the rest of the story or release, which presents increasingly fine detail. Editors can cut the story at almost any point and still have a piece that makes sense.

In reporting news, journalists traditionally are told to remember the five Ws and an H: who, what, where, when, why, and how. For a story on research results, the "who" would include who did the research and, if rel-

II. Preparing the Piece

evant, who funded it. The "what" would include what was studied and what the findings were. The "where" would include the institution where the research was done and the journal or conference where it was published or presented. The "when" could include the date of publication or presentation. The "why" could include why the research was done and why the findings may be important, as well as the likely mechanism behind what was observed. Part of the "how" would be how the research was done. Another part would be how the findings fit with those of other studies—in other words, the context for the findings.

News stories reporting results of biomedical research often have failed to provide such context. For example, those on studies suggesting that given factors affect the likelihood of developing types of cancer have commonly reported the findings in isolation, rather than as part of an often complex big picture (Mann 1995). As emphasized elsewhere, such context is crucial to health writing that is accurate in the fullest sense and is the most helpful.

Context is one area considered in an index of scientific quality that researchers at McMaster University in Canada developed for evaluating

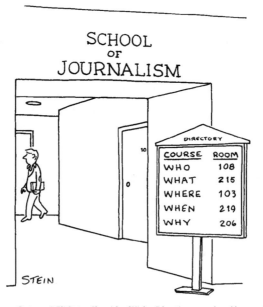

Cartoon © Eli Stein, *Chronicle of Higher Education,* reproduced by permission.

health-related news reports. As noted by the researchers, this index, consisting of eight questions, can serve as a checklist for health writers. The questions, as stated by the researchers, are:

(1) Is it clear to whom the information in the report applies (i.e. to which population the evidence is applicable)?
(2) Are facts clearly distinguished from opinions?
(3) Is the assessment of the credibility (validity) of the evidence clear and well-founded (not misleading)?
(4) Is the strength or magnitude of the findings (effects, risks, or costs) that are the main focus of the article clearly reported?
(5) Is there a clear and well-founded (not misleading) assessment of the precision of any estimates that are reported or of the probability that any of the reported findings might be due to chance?
(6) Is the consistency of the evidence (between studies) considered and is the assessment well-founded (not misleading)?
(7) Are all of the important consequences (benefits, risks and costs) of concern relative to the central topic of the report identified?
(8) Based on your answers to the above questions, how would you rate the overall scientific quality of the report? (Oxman et al. 1993)

Consider consulting this list when you write news stories or news releases on research.

As well as being suitably structured and containing suitable information, a news story or news release must be readable. And to fulfill its role of attracting media coverage, a news release must indicate whom to contact for further information. A British study (Albert 1995) suggests that many news releases are impenetrably written or fail to state whom to contact. In preparing news stories and releases, as in other health writing, attention to the audience remains crucial.

FRANK & ERNEST® by Bob Thaves

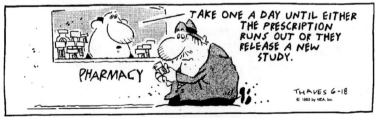

With permission of Bob Thaves.

II. Preparing the Piece

Figures 8-3 through 8-5 present three examples: a radio story reporting research findings, a newspaper story announcing approval of a drug, and a news release about a diagnostic test. Comments on content and technique accompany each example, reinforcing points made above and elsewhere in the book.

Investigative and Depth Reporting

What? A separate section on investigative and depth reporting? Isn't a major message of this book that all health writing should draw on thorough investigation? True, but some types of health writing entail particularly deep, broad, or ingenious investigation. Among them are stories that seek to uncover problems in health care and those that discern, describe, and interpret broad trends with implications for health. These types of health writing are the focus of this section.

Many of us enter health writing partly because we have high regard for medical research and health care and enjoy reporting favorable news such as medical advances. However, medicine also has a sorrier side, and documenting and publicizing problems in realms such as health care can help lead to their solution. Given the scope of work that may be required, a team approach can be a good option, with the health writer lending knowledge of medical topics, sources, and institutions and a journalist experienced in investigative reporting bringing attitudes and approaches from that realm.

Among areas for possible investigation are the functioning of medical institutions, the competence of health practitioners, the costs and financing of health care, the efficacy and safety of drugs and medical devices, and the prevalence of occupational and environmental diseases. Are there problems in the performance of health care facilities, clinical laboratories, nursing homes, home health care services, or the like? Is local emergency medical care failing to meet standards? Are nonprofit institutions such as health-related associations making inappropriate use of funds? Are given practitioners endangering public well-being by providing health care without appropriate competence or credentials? Are medical devices or drugs with substantial problems remaining available? Are there sites where high rates of occupational or environmental disease are not being suitably addressed?

If so, you may have the start of an investigative story or series. At a recent conference on investigative reporting, one reporter told of exposing a fertility clinic that was illicitly giving women other women's eggs. Another recounted uncovering the case of a heart transplant program that was no longer doing transplants—and yet was still accepting patients. A third reporter told of investigating a doctor who was doing unnecessary medical procedures—and doing them incompetently.

Figure 8-3:   News Story, "Smoking and Breast Cancer May Be Linked, Study Shows," Morning Edition (National Public Radio), April 26, 1996

Story	*Comments*
Alex Chadwick, Host: . . . A new study raises the possibility that many cases of breast cancer may be caused by smoking, or by breathing secondhand tobacco smoke. This study seemingly contradicts dozens of others that have shown no link between these major public-health issues, but experts say there are compelling reasons not to ignore this study as a fluke. Instead, the conflicting conclusions should spur more study into the potential connection between increasing breast-cancer rates and tobacco use. NPR's Richard Harris has the story.	"Summary lead": overview of study's main finding (note that uncertainty is acknowledged) Context: comparison with findings of other studies Continuing overview of the main points of the story
Richard Harris, Reporter: More than 20 studies have looked for a connection between cigarette smoking and breast cancer without finding a strong connection. But Alfredo Morabia from the University Hospital in Geneva, Switzerland, says all those studies have made a big assumption he didn't agree with—that is, women exposed to secondhand smoke were still considered to be nonsmokers.	Context: previous studies Who": the researcher "Where": his affiliation "How": way in which this study's approach differed from that of previous studies
Alfredo Morabia, University Hospi-	Words of researcher himself

Figure 8-3:   News Story (*continued*)

Story	*Comments*
tal, Geneva, Switzerland: So we performed the first study in which we could separate women that were really never exposed to tobacco smoke from women who had been exposed passively.	
Richard Harris: And what he found was startling, as he reports in the *American Journal of Epidemiology's* May 1st issue—smoking women were indeed at significantly greater risk of breast cancer. Their risk was doubled or tripled when compared with women who reported no significant exposure to tobacco smoke. Even more surprising was that women who breathed a lot of secondhand smoke during their lifetimes also had a high risk of breast cancer, compared with the non-exposed women.	"Where": site of publication of the study "When": date of publication Mention of statistical significance; inclusion of numbers Use of "surprising" here and "startling" above helps attract audience's attention to key findings
Alfredo Morabia: We weren't expecting that. We thought that passive smoking would be considered with a weaker risk than active smoking, but that's not what we found.	Reinforcement by the researcher
Richard Harris: In other smoking-related diseases higher doses of tobacco smoke mean higher risks, so active smokers are usually at much higher risk than people who breathe secondhand smoke. Julie Palmer at Boston University says these findings really stand out. Taken literally, this study suggests smoking and passive smoke could cause more breast cancer than any other known risk factor.	Context: contrast with somewhat analogous findings Opinion by expert not associated with the study "Why": importance of the study (impact if findings are true)
Julie Palmer, Boston University: This was really a shockingly high effect or estimate of effect, and it would	Comment by outside expert

Figure 8-3: (*continued*)

Story	*Comments*
probably lead most people to discount these results.	
Richard Harris: But Palmer says the study itself has no obvious glaring flaws, so it's a finding that can't simply be dismissed as a fluke. But Morabia will have to find a way to explain why much lower doses of secondhand smoke appear to be almost as dangerous as huge doses of carcinogens from active smoking. He theorizes that poisons from cigarette smoke build up in fatty breast tissue of susceptible women, and it doesn't take all that much to trigger breast cancer. But he hasn't proven that. Most important, Morabia acknowledges other scientists will have to carry out similar studies and come up with similar results.	Expert opinion on the study design and whether to take the results seriously

"Why": question of mechanism behind the findings

"Why": researcher's speculation on the mechanism

Distinction of speculation from established findings

Need for confirmation in order to accept findings |
| Alfredo Morabia: One study is not enough to say, "Well, there is a causal relationship, we have to bring this message to the population." But one study like ours is enough to say that there may be something, and we need to take this very seriously because it may lead to simple public-health information to the women and to reduction of the number of cancer[s] in the population. | Idea well expressed by researcher

Possible public-health implications |
| Richard Harris: If his conclusion holds up, he says it could explain a sizable fraction of breast cancer in the United States. So, considering the huge amount of attention being paid to both tobacco and breast cancer right now, this is a question that's not likely to languish. This is Richard Harris in Washington. | Possible public-health implications

Reference to newsworthiness of topic

Allusion to likely future research |

Story	*Comments*
A drug derived from the bark of a Chinese tree was approved by the Food and Drug Administration on Wednesday to help women whose ovarian cancer has progressed despite other treatments.	"Summary lead": announcement of new drug's approval; indication of the drug's use
Topotecan is the first of a new class of cancer drugs that inhibit an enzyme essential for growth of tumors. It appears to work at least as well as the widely used ovarian cancer therapy Taxol.	Newness: novelty of the drug's mechanism of action Context: comparison with effectiveness of a previously approved drug
While doctors caution that it's not a breakthrough, FDA Commissioner David Kessler said topotecan "is an important option" for advanced patients.	Caution: limitation of the drug's importance Statement by authority
Manufactured by SmithKline Beecham Pharmaceuticals, topotecan will be sold under the name Hycamtin and will begin sales in several weeks.	"Who": manufacturer of the drug Trade name of the drug "When": time sales will begin
Ovarian cancer strikes about 26,700 American women every year and kills about 14,800.	Background: incidence and mortality of condition
In a study of 337 women, topotecan helped shrink the tumors of 17 percent of patients, a response rate comparable to that experienced by patients taking Taxol, the FDA said.	The inverted pyramid continues: statistics on effectiveness of drug; more detailed comparison with established drug
The study found no statistically significant difference in survival between patients taking topotecan and those taking Taxol.	Mention of statistical significance
SmithKline touted data that suggested topotecan stopped ovarian tumors from progressing for 23 weeks vs. 14 weeks for Taxol patients.	Possible advantage noted by manufacturer
However, topotecan patients experienced somewhat more severe side effects, particularly a drop in their immune system's ability to fight infections. This side effect is treatable,	Side effects

Figure 8-4: *(continued)*

Story

although some women may require
hospitalization.

The FDA approved topotecan as a
second-line therapy, to be offered as an
option for patients after another treatment has failed.

"I don't think we can say with certainty yet whether it's better than
Taxol," cautioned FDA oncology director Dr. Robert DeLay. "We simply don't
have enough data to address the question. . . . And they may turn out to be
complementary drugs, so the question
of better may not be an issue."

Indeed, scientists are intrigued by
topotecan because it works differently
than other cancer drugs.

Whenever a new class of medicines
is discovered, one hope is that combin-
ing it with older drugs could deal tu-
mors a one-two punch.

Topotecan inhibits an enzyme
called topoisomerase-I that is important for tumor growth. Existing drugs
have proved beneficial against some
cancers by attacking a related enzyme,
topoisomerase-II.

The National Cancer Institute and
SmithKline are studying whether com-
bining these two types of drugs could
help certain patients.

Also, tests of topotecan as a first-
line therapy for small-cell lung cancer
have found response rates as high as 39
percent, the NCI said.

Topotecan was discovered in the
bark of a Chinese tree called *Camp-
totheca acuminata.*

The tree, as well as a relative that
harbors the ingredient, is common and
fast-growing, so SmithKline said
topotecan's supply is plentiful.

Comments

The inverted pyramid continues: more
detail on approved use of the drug

Quote by expert

Limitations of available information

Transition

Background: general strategy for using
such drugs

The inverted pyramid continues: more
detailed description of the drug mechanism

Context: related mechanism of some
other drugs

Ongoing studies

Studies suggesting drug's usefulness in
a related condition

Background: origin of drug

Adequacy of natural supply of drug

Figure 8-5: News Release, " 'Ultrafast CT' with Electron Beam Accurately Predicts Heart Attacks in Seemingly Healthy People, Study Shows," American Heart Association, June 1, 1996

Story	*Comments*
"Ultrafast CT" scanning with an electron beam proved many times more powerful than the best available non-invasive test in predicting heart attacks and other coronary disease episodes, even in apparently healthy people, a new study shows.	"Summary lead": overview of findings
By measuring the amount of calcium deposits that build up in coronaries—in a disease process commonly called hardening of the arteries—ultrafast CT accurately predicts cardiovascular disease events in people with no symptoms, doctors at St. Francis Hospital in Roslyn, N.Y., report in today's (June 1) American Heart Association journal *Circulation*.	"How": what the test measures Link to a familiar concept "Who": affiliation of researchers "When": publication date "Where": publication site
"This is the first large, written report with a high degree of completeness of follow-up (99.8%) documenting the prospective short-term predictive value of EBCT (electron beam computed tomography) of the coronary arteries in asymptomatic patients," the team writes.	Newness of findings Indicators of quality of study (size, completeness of follow-up, prospective design) Delay in use of technical term for the test until the main news has been presented
EBCT is a "tool that allows us to identify people who are at high risk for coronary disease," says Yadon Arad, M.D., the study's lead investigator and director of preventive cardiology at St. Francis Hospital. "EBCT screening would enable me to identify individuals in the early stages of coronary disease who would benefit the most from therapies (such as drug treatments, diet and exercise) that might prevent heart attacks."	Quote from, and title of, study's lead investigator Practical implications of the findings
EBCT scanning costs from $375 to $500 in the United States, which is	Cost of the testing

1 0 8

Figure 8-5:   (*continued*)

Story	*Comments*
"relatively inexpensive, compared to other diagnostic tests in cardiology," he says.	Context: comparison with costs of other tests
The researchers used EBCT in 1,173 asymptomatic patients between September 1993 and March 1994 and then followed the patients for an average of 19 months. During the follow-up, 18 patients had a total of 26 cardiovascular events—including one death, seven heart attacks, eight coronary bypass surgeries, nine coronary angioplasties and one stroke.	The inverted pyramid continues: more detailed description of the study
"We conclude that EBCT-based screening for coronary artery disease shows great applicability to the development of cardiovascular disease events in a relatively short time period (average, 19 months) in a mostly middle-aged group that was 71 percent male," the investigators write in *Circulation*.	Nature of the group studied (and thus implications for generalizability)
But Lewis Wexler, M.D., of Stanford University Medical Center in California, cautions that EBCT scanning is still undergoing clinical investigation. "As promising as the results of the study appear to be, it's still an experimental screening technique," he says.	Caution: statement by outside expert that the testing still is experimental
"Large-scale prospective studies are needed to prove its predictive value, which will differ depending on a patient's age, gender and the presence of coronary artery disease risk factors."	Need for further research
Wexler chairs an AHA panel that is developing a scientific statement on coronary calcification and EBCT.	Mention of organization issuing the news release
Alan Guerci, M.D., study senior author and director of research at St. Francis Hospital, says: "Our study shows that EBCT scanning of the coronary arteries has a predictive accuracy	The inverted pyramid continues: more detailed quantification of the results of the study

Figure 8-5:   **News Release (*continued*)**

Story

that exceeds by a large margin that of
any other non-invasive technology."

Although cholesterol testing involves drawing a blood sample, it's
considered to be non-invasive, Guerci
notes. But even the best cholesterol test
(the ratio of total cholesterol to "good"
HDL cholesterol) achieves an "odds ratio" of only about 1.6, he says. (An
odds ratio of 1 implies no increased
risk.) Guerci defines odds ratio as "the
probability of getting sick or dying if
your test result is abnormal, divided by
the probability of something bad hap-
pening to you if your test is normal."

His team found EBCT achieved
odds ratios ranging from 20 to 35,
making the scanning technique more
than 10 times more powerful a predic-
tor of coronary disease episodes than
cholesterol testing, he says.

Autopsy reports and other data
have consistently shown a correlation
between coronary artery calcium content (CAC) and the severity of coronary artery disease, the authors note.
EBCT provides doctors a CAC "score"
for each patient based on the amount
of calcium seen in the scans. Among
study participants, CAC scores averaging 935 in patients with coronary
events, vs. scores averaging 144 in patients without events. And those individuals with a CAC score above 160
had a 35-fold higher risk of developing
a coronary event than those with
scores below 160, the researchers
found.

While this is the first published report of a follow-up of apparently
healthy persons undergoing EBCT
scanning of the heart, three other stud-

Comments

Explanation of statistical concept

"Why": rationale for expecting that the
testing would work

Further quantification of findings

Context: other more-preliminary studies
with similar findings

Figure 8-5: *(continued)*

Story	*Comments*
ies presented at two recent AHA scientific meetings had similar findings, Guerci points out. "Now there are four studies with a total of 2,745 asymptomatic patients and all four show the coronary calcium score is highly predictive of future cardiac events."	Mention again of the organization issuing the release
Because the coronary arteries supply blood to the cardiac muscle and are in constant motion as the heart beats, obtaining X-ray images of the moving vessels was difficult until the new superfast machines were built. Ultrafast CT devices using electron beams now are available in about 25 cities in the United States and about 30 cities in Europe and Asia.	"Why": reason the new technique is needed to obtain the findings

Availability of the equipment |
Guerci emphasizes there's no link between calcium deposits in the coronary arteries and calcium-rich foods, or the calcium supplements taken by many older women. These women have a high risk of osteoporosis and "they should not lower their calcium intake because of ourfindings," he says.	Anticipation and countering of a possible misinterpretation of the findings' implications
Other co-authors with Arad and Guerci are Louise A. Spadaro, M.D.; Ken Goodman, M.D; Alfonso Lledo-Perez, M.D.; Scott Sherman, M.D., and Gail Lerner, M.S.	The inverted pyramid continues: names of co-authors
Circulation is one of five scientific journals published by the Dallas-based AHA.	Sponsorship of the journal; mention again of the organization issuing the release

Two sources of detailed guidance in uncovering, documenting, and reporting such problems are the recent editions of *The Reporter's Handbook: An Investigator's Guide to Documents and Techniques* (Ullmann and Colbert 1991, Weinberg 1996). Each of these two editions not only supplies extensive overall guidance in investigative reporting but also has a chapter on investigative reporting on health care. Because the two editions differ in areas emphasized, consulting both can be worthwhile. Another poten-

II. Preparing the Piece

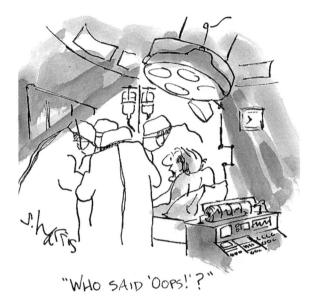

"WHO SAID 'OOPS!'?"

© Sidney Harris, reproduced by permission.

tially useful book is *Investigative Reporting for Print and Broadcast* (Gaines 1994), which also contains a chapter on investigating health care.

The organization under which *The Reporter's Handbook* was prepared, Investigative Reporters and Editors (IRE), also offers other resources useful in investigative reporting on health care. Through the IRE Resource Center, copies of investigative stories from various print and broadcast media can be obtained; a recent search disclosed more than 200 such stories available on topics in health care. Reading the stories obtained on one's subject can suggest ways of gathering information and presenting it, and consulting those who prepared the stories can yield additional guidance. Among other items available from the resource center are handouts from IRE conferences, which often include sessions on aspects of investigative health reporting. Further information on IRE and its services can be obtained from Investigative Reporters and Editors, 138 Neff Annex, Missouri School of Journalism, Columbia, Missouri 65211, phone (573) 882-2042, fax (573) 882-5431, e-mail jourire@muccmail.missouri.edu. The IRE Web site is http://www.ire.org.

Depth or investigative reporting also may focus on epidemiologic and other trends affecting health. One example is the Pulitzer-Prize-winning series "When Bugs Fight Back" by science and medical writer Mike Toner of the *Atlanta Journal-Constitution*. Drawing on many sources, this extensive series addresses two parallel developments: the increasing resistance of microorganisms to antibiotics, and the increasing resistance of insects and weeds to pesticides. A booklet containing the series may be obtained from the *Journal-Constitution,* and excerpts from the series appear in the anthology *The New Science Journalists* (Anton and McCourt 1995).

Personal and social dimensions of illness also can be areas for health writing in depth. Two highly lauded examples, each dealing with AIDS in a rural setting, are the newspaper series "AIDS in the Heartland" (Banaszynski and Pieri 1987-88) and the book *My Own Country: A Doctor's Story* (Verghese 1994).

Health writing in depth can include going beyond individual incidences of disease or injury to seek broader patterns and thus possible means of prevention. In one such case of reporter-as-epidemiologist, a correspondent obtained government records on snowmobile fatalities. Among the findings his analysis disclosed was a strong association with high blood alcohol levels (Imrie 1996).

Investigative and depth reporting typically entail much time and effort. It is wise to think about whether a given project deserves the investment, or whether the resources would be better devoted to one or more other stories. Among aspects to consider are the importance of the problem or issue to public health, the potential of the project to enlighten the audience about its world, and the potential of the reporting to stimulate action that would benefit health. Factors affecting the likelihood that such reporting will influence health policy have begun to be explored through case studies (Walsh-Childers 1994a). Among factors that seemed to contribute to one series' success in spurring policy changes were agreement among experts regarding solutions, support by private citizen groups and public officials, the location of the newspaper in the capital city, widespread distribution of reprints, follow-up reporting on the issue, and publicity when the series won a Pulitzer Prize (Walsh-Childers 1994b).

The Feature Article Family

Just as what's new and what's wrong are only parts of the world of health, news reporting and investigative reporting are not all of health writing. Many aspects of the world of health are best conveyed through feature articles, which tend to be well suited for integrating information on a topic and showing how matters evolve.

II. Preparing the Piece

This section deals with articles in the feature article family—among them, overview articles, narratives, and profiles. Although these types of feature are dealt with individually, it should be noted that many articles are hybrids.

Overview pieces acquaint an audience with a topic such as a given disease (or group of diseases), a diagnostic technique or treatment, or the functioning of a part of the body. A staple of magazines and newsletters, such pieces also appear in such forms as patient-education brochures, encyclopedia entries, and sidebars to news stories. In an overview article on a disease or other condition, key medical content to present typically includes the definition of the condition, the manifestations, the causative agent, the disease mechanism, the epidemiology of the condition (that is, its pattern of distribution within the population), means of diagnosis, means of treatment, prognosis, and prevention. In addition, historical, economic, ethical, and social perspectives can be worth providing, and items such as literary references can enrich the piece. Often, listing sources of further information also is worthwhile.

Figure 8.7 presents an example of a brief but informative overview on sleepwalking drawn from a broader piece on physician-writer John Stone's experience as a sleepwalker. Noted alongside the example are types of information presented. Also noted are some aspects of the writing technique, as well as other items relating to material discussed elsewhere in this book.

A feature format that can work very well for health writing is that of the narrative, or tale. Such a narrative may recount a surgical operation, trace a patient's experience with a major illness or injury, follow the probings of a biomedical researcher, or describe the solution of a puzzling case or outbreak. As stories, such accounts tend to be highly engaging, and they can serve as frameworks for memorably presenting considerable amounts of information obtained from various written and other sources. They are particularly well geared for illustrating medical thinking and showing the process, rather than only the products, of biomedical investigation.

One outstanding example of a medical narrative is the Pulitzer-Prize-winning "Mrs. Kelly's Monster" by Jon Franklin. This story about a brain operation has been reprinted in annotated form (Franklin 1986, 216-35; Friedman, Dunwoody, and Rogers 1986, 271-84), with the writer explaining his use of various literary techniques. Reading the annotated version can be highly instructive not only in crafting narratives, but more broadly in writing effectively about medical topics.

Many tales of puzzling cases or outbreaks and their solution also are

Figure 8-7: Overview on Sleepwalking, from "Night Wanderings" by John Stone, *New York Times Magazine*, January 19, 1992, pp. 14, 16

Story	*Comments*
[opening series of paragraphs in which the author, a physician, discusses the sleepwalking he has experienced since his wife's recent death and mentions the sleepwalking and sleeptalking he did in his youth]	
Like most physicians, I have a certain hesitation in searching the dispassionate "medical literature" for insights into my own maladies. This is especially true for problems outside my area of expertise, as this sleep disorder is for me. What if I were to learn that the abrupt onset of sleepwalking is often an early sign of a brain tumor? But eventually I did go and ask the reference librarian for her help. She came through with wonderful information that I began to sift with the physician part of my brain.	Transition into overview of topic (Note: Mention of the literature can be a good transitional device in such circumstances) (Note consultation of reference librarian, in keeping with guidance in this book)
By definition, *sleepwalking* is a sequence of complex behaviors that begin (usually) during the first third or so of an otherwise good night's sleep. It turns out to be most common in children, 15 percent of whom sleepwalk at some point. It seems to be much less common, even rare, in adults.	Definition Information on epidemiology
But the true frequency of somnambulism is difficult to be sure about because we walkers don't remember our shuffles. The development of "sleep labs" (in which brain waves, heart rate and other measurements are done during sleep) has helped. Sleepwalking in adults generally appears as a response to stress. With the cataclysmic loss of my wife, I qualify for that diagnosis: we had been married almost 33 years.	Limitations of available data Gentle introduction of technical term (meaning is clear from context) A causative factor Use of example to provide support
Sleep-*talking*, such as I did about Margaret, is apparently pretty uncommon. And the words spoken at such times are often hard to understand. In-	Lighter paragraph—helps keep overview from becoming too dry

Figure 8-7: **Overview (*continued*)**

Story	*Comments*
cidentally, the delightful medical name for talking in one's sleep is *somniloquy*. Done alone, as it most certainly is, I suppose it's a somniloquy soliloquy.	Word play
Which reminds me of W. H. Auden's definition of a *professor* as "one who talks in someone else's sleep."	Literary reference/ Lively quotation
The experts divide sleepwalking into two types. The first consists of passive behavior without attendant fear.	Summary before details
For example, one woman removed all her shoes from her closet and lined them up on the windowsill. A medical student who came by my office just now tells me that she used to walk in her sleep when she was a child; she would be discovered by her father in the kitchen setting the table for breakfast or going out at midnight in search of the morning paper. Incidentally, vision seems to be intact in sleepwalkers, so she could have found the paper, had it been there.	Use of examples or anecdotes to clarify abstract material, engage audience, make the content more memorable
In the second type of sleepwalking, self-injury or even violence can occur. Such episodes may begin with a terrified (and terrifying) shriek, accompanied by the rapid heart rate of fear, a kind of "night terror"; the walker will sometimes lash out obliviously and strike the bed partner with the fist. Self-injury is a potential danger, too; in one study, a patient walked out on the window ledge of his apartment, which happened to be on the 35th floor.	Transition Example Example or anecdote; note how author builds up to the "punch line"
Treatment of sleepwalking seems to be highly variable: tranquilizers, antidepressants, psychotherapy, hypnosis and behavioral therapy have all been tried. So have acupuncture and herbal medicines. . . .	Information on treatment
[closing series of paragraphs, in which the author further discusses his own sleepwalking and reflects on its meaning]	

available as models. Some of the classics are by Berton Roueché, whose medical mystery nonfiction appeared in *The New Yorker* over several decades and has been collected in several volumes (for example, Roueché 1982, Roueché 1986, Roueché 1995). More recently, many well-crafted, informative medical narratives have appeared in the "Vital Signs" section of *Discover* magazine. As well as illustrating their genre, these accounts demonstrate various general aspects of good health-writing technique. In addition, reading them can readily increase a health writer's medical knowledge.

Profiles of people also can be engaging vehicles for presenting material from the world of health. Profiles work well for portraying process—whether of living with a disease, doing biomedical research, treating patients, or seeking to influence health policy. And of course they inherently contain human interest. One caution, though: Beware of presenting stereotypes, such as the selfless health-care provider, the single-minded researcher, the pitiful person with a disability, or the person totally undaunted thereby. Put aside preconceptions, listen to and observe the people you are portraying, and present them in realistic complexity.

To prepare a well-rounded profile, draw on varied sources. Before interviewing, look at the subject's resume or curriculum vitae if one exists. Also look at other background material, such as articles by researchers and news releases on their work, or overview pieces on an individual's disease. As well as noting what the subject says when interviewed, observe the subject and his or her environment. Consider interviewing the subject more than once, perhaps in different settings such as work and home. Maybe observe the subject in action. For "reflected light," interview people who know the person being profiled. And even if you are not the photographer for the story, consider taking photos to refer to when writing the piece.

Other types of feature stories for health writers to consider are service, how-to, and personal-experience articles. Service articles give consumers information on products, services, or facilities, often to aid in choosing among them; how-to and personal-experience articles are just what their name says. Service and how-to articles, which often overlap, need thorough information-gathering and organized presentation, often through devices such as lists, charts, and diagrams. For personal-experience articles, the point is to use your experience or that of another person as a vehicle for conveying information and insight, not as a forum for showing off scars or for griping.

"I do think I know what these night wanderings are all about in my own life . . ." is how Stone ends his combination of personal-experience piece and overview article on sleepwalking. If you, like Stone, have written a health feature well, readers will reach the end not only with more information but also with greater understanding.

Other Genres

Other genres also are open to health writers. Among them are columns, book reviews, and—yes—obituaries.

Health columns have long been popular with the public. They are a venue particularly open to health writers with backgrounds as health professionals. Some questions to address when thinking of embarking on a column are how broad or narrow the scope should be, what format to use (question-and-answer or essay), and whether to have another writer collaborate. Also before embarking, consider whether you really have the material—and the time—to turn out column after column.

Book reviewing is another option. Given the popularity of publications on health, books to review abound. If you have read this health writer's handbook, you should have a good start at evaluating writing on health. In addition, lists of items to consider discussing in a review (for example, Gastel 1991) are available. Although reviewing books rarely pays well, it provides opportunity for thorough and thoughtful reading and sometimes for relatively ready publication in otherwise highly competitive sites. Plus, normally you get to keep the book.

Finally, obituaries of health professionals and researchers are an additional form of health writing—one that health writers at institutions may be called on to do. Items typically included are the individual's most recent professional position held, education, professional accomplishments, and survivors. Some of the best obituaries are essentially profiles, drawing both on written sources and on interviews with individuals such as colleagues.

As a health writer, you may also have opportunities to write material in other genres—such as editorials and humor pieces. Now, having considered some of the main genres, you may more easily analyze pieces in others and model your writing accordingly. And so with obituaries this chapter ends.

ʃƐNʃITIVITY ɅND ʃTYLƐ

You have gathered your information and organized it. You know how to present it clearly and engagingly. But as you write, concerns arise. How can you refer to people with disabilities or diseases sensitively and without offense? Are you using health-related terms correctly? What about other matters of usage? The current chapter addresses such questions. First it provides guidance in writing about people with disabilities or diseases. Then it focuses on some basic matters of medical usage. Finally, it deals with some general items of usage that often arise in health writing.

When additional questions arise, consulting general and medical style manuals can be helpful. A standard style manual for newspaper writing, and also a good resource for writing for other media, is *The Associated Press Stylebook and Libel Manual* (Goldstein 1996). Among the many entries in this alphabetically organized manual are some relating specifically to medicine or health. For medical writing, a basic resource is the *American Medical Association Manual of Style* (Iverson et al. 1989; 1998). Although this manual is geared mainly to writing for medical journals, much of its material on usage and related subjects also applies to popular medical writing. Consider keeping such manuals at your desk.

Writing about People with Disabilities or Diseases

Some years ago an older colleague mentioned having trained at a facility called the Hospital for the Ruptured and Crippled. Today, such insensitive phrasing is rare. But how to write most suitably about people with disabilities or diseases remains partially unresolved.

Guidelines continue to evolve, and preferences sometimes differ among groups or individuals. However, the following suggestions, drawn from one or more sources (American Psychological Association 1994, Disabilities Committee of the American Society of Newspaper Editors 1990, Knatterud 1991, Maggio 1991, National Easter Seal Society n.d., Research

II. Preparing the Piece

and Training Center on Independent Living 1993, Schwartz et al. 1995), can at least provide a useful starting point.

(1) Check preferences of people being portrayed. Different people prefer different terms for their conditions. For example, some people with dwarfism wish to be called "people of short stature"; others favor "little people." Find out what terminology people prefer, and if possible use it in your story.

(2) Obtain guidance from relevant associations and from editors. Associations dealing with particular diseases or conditions often devote considerable attention to identifying acceptable terminology. Check with these associations, or see what wording they use in their publications. Likewise check with editors for whom you are preparing pieces; the publications or institutions for which they work may have guidelines regarding which terms to use.

(3) Avoid labels that negate individuality. People are individuals, regardless of whether they have a disability or disease in common. Thus, avoid terms such as "the disabled," "the retarded," "a diabetic," or "an arthritic." Such terms tend to obliterate individuality and may promote the development or perpetuation of stereotypes. In short, they are dehumanizing.

(4) Emphasize "people"; try to put "people" first. Instead of terms such as those above, choose wordings that include "people" or the like. And if possible put "people" or the equivalent first, especially on initial mention. For example, speak of "people with disabilities" or "a woman with diabetes." For conciseness and crispness in later mentions, condensed versions such as "blind people" or "stroke survivors" may be acceptable.

(5) Do not confuse "disability" and "handicap." A disability is a condition that interferes with one or more major life activities, such as walking, hearing, breathing, or learning. In contrast, a handicap is something that is a barrier to a person with a disability. For example, a man whose legs are paralyzed has a disability, not a handicap. However, stairs may be a handicap to him, as may the attitudes of some employers.

(6) Do not refer to people merely as "disabled." People may have one or more disabilities, but no one is totally disabled. Rather than calling a person disabled, write that the person has a disability (or disabilities). Probably better, indicate the nature of the condition.

(7) Avoid melodramatic wording. Do not use language such as "afflicted with," "crippled by," "stricken with," "suffering from," or "victim of." Simply say that the person has AIDS or multiple sclerosis or lung cancer; if relevant, show how the condition has affected the person's life. Doing so will convey the needed information without over-dramatizing the situation, implying passivity, or inadvertently diminishing the person's dignity.

(8) Present wheelchairs and other aids as enabling, not confining. Such aids help free people from limitations associated with their disabilities, rather

than serving as constraints. Thus, do not use language such as "confined to a wheelchair" or "wheelchair-bound." Rather, say that a person "uses a wheelchair."

(9) Call people "patients" only in the context of medical treatment. "Patient" is not synonymous with a person who has a disability or disease. Call people "patients" only when discussing their medical care.

(10) Beware of referring to people as "dying of." Reserve such wording for those close to the time of death. Do not say that people are dying of AIDS or cancer or emphysema when in fact they are living with the condition.

(11) Avoid referring to people without a given disability or disease as "normal" or "able-bodied." People without a given condition are not necessarily functioning well and healthy in all regards. Nor does having a disability, as most of us eventually do to some extent, render someone outside the norm. Here, as elsewhere, be precise. For example, say "people with normal heart function" or "people without hearing impairments." Likewise, rather than saying that one child in a family has arthritis but the other is normal, say that the one child has arthritis but the other does not.

(12) Consider whether you would be comfortable with the writing if you had the condition being discussed. If the content or language makes you uneasy, think again. Reflect on what seems insensitive and how it might be remedied. If in doubt, return to the beginning of this list and request outside guidance.

Additional guidance also is available in two brief but substantive brochures: *Guidelines for Reporting and Writing about People with Disabilities* (1993), published by the Research and Training Center on Independent Living (4089 Dole Building, University of Kansas, Lawrence, Kansas 66045, telephone (913) 864-4095, fax (913) 864-5063), and *Awareness is the First Step Towards Change: Tips for Portraying People with Disabilities in the Media* (n.d.), published by the National Easter Seal Society (230 West Monroe Street, Suite 1800, Chicago, Illinois 60606, telephone (312) 726-6200, fax (312) 726-1494). As well as containing general advice on wording, the former includes definitions and preferred wordings relating to various types of disability, and the latter presents tips on interviewing people with disabilities.

Some Matters of Medical Usage

Is it better to say that someone is "a woman" or "a female"? Should names of medications be capitalized? And are life span and life expectancy the same? Health writers often face such questions. Here are answers regarding some matters of medical usage.

II. Preparing the Piece

Acute and Chronic; Serious and Severe

An acute condition is one of sudden onset and limited duration; a chronic condition is one that lasts a long time. Calling a condition "acute" says nothing about its seriousness. A heart attack can be acute, but so can indigestion.

And speaking of seriousness, "serious" and "severe" do not mean the same thing. A condition can be severe—that is, have especially powerful manifestations—without being particularly serious. Think about a severe cold.

Age and Gender

How old can one be and still be called a "girl" or "boy"? What age range does "youth" encompass? At what age should one be termed an "older person"? Authorities disagree on such matters. And even if they agreed, members of the public would interpret the terms differently. The solution is to specify the age group. Say that subjects ranged in age from 18 to 24 years, or that side effects were more common in patients above age 80. Also, beware of referring to age when something more specific is meant; if you mean frail, say frail, not old.

As for gender: When possible, refer to people as "men" or "women," "boys" or "girls." Try to avoid the terms "males" and "females," which tend to be dehumanizing and generally should be reserved for lab rats. Use these terms for people only when no other wording is feasible, such as when a population consists of people of both genders and unknown age.

Attribution to a Journal

People sometimes write, "The *New England Journal of Medicine* says . . ." or "*JAMA* reported . . ." But except perhaps in editorials, journals themselves do not make statements. Rather, as noted earlier in this book, they publish researchers' articles that the editors view as having sufficient merit. Such publication means that the editors consider the work sufficiently strong and important, but it is not an endorsement of the conclusions as true. Given the preliminary or otherwise limited nature of much research, such endorsement often cannot be validly given. More accurate wordings include, "An article in the *New England Journal of Medicine* says . . ." and "Authors of a study published in *JAMA* reported . . ."

9.   Sensitivity and Style

Breakthroughs

In general, avoid using the word "breakthrough," which suggests that progress in medical research occurs in sudden large leaps. Major advances in medicine typically reflect long, slow progress. Unless an advance is one of the rare exceptions, do not term it a "breakthrough." Instead, use words such as "advance" or "development." Also, if possible, portray the work that led to the discovery or innovation.

Capitalization of Disease Names

A common error is to capitalize disease names—to write of Multiple Sclerosis or Lupus or Mononucleosis. Only those parts of disease names that are derived from proper nouns, such as names of people or places, should be capitalized. Thus, "Down syndrome" (or, in some renderings, "Down's syndrome"), named after English physician John Down; and "Lyme disease," named after Lyme, Connecticut. Speaking of disease names, make sure they are properly spelled. Do not be like the young journalist who wrote of "Lyme's disease"—or the editor who failed to check whether this name was correct.

Case versus Patient

Use "patient"—not "case," which is dehumanizing—to refer to a person receiving medical attention. A patient is a person; a case is an instance (for example, of a disease). Thus, use "case" only where "instance" could also be used. You can say that in 12 cases (instances), a side effect developed. However, you must say that 12 patients (not cases, as you are referring to people) developed the side effect.

Degrees and Titles

Health professionals and researchers have a wide variety of academic degrees. If you write for a publication that lists degrees, be sure to state each person's degree, or degrees, correctly. Do not assume that a medical doctor necessarily has an MD degree. Some medical doctors have DO (doctor of osteopathy) degrees; doctors educated in countries where medical education begins immediately after high school sometimes have MB (bachelor of medicine) or other degrees.

II.   Preparing the Piece

Publications differ in their policies on use of the title "Dr." Some use it for people with all types of doctorates: PhD, MD, and other. Others restrict it to medical doctors. Find out the policy of the publication for which you are writing, double-check the degrees of the people, and proceed accordingly.

Some publications use people's degrees on first mention and their titles thereafter. For example, they may introduce a doctor as "Naomi F. Singer, MD" and refer to her later as "Dr. Singer." Avoid redundant wording such as "Dr. Singer, MD."

"Die of"

In conversation, it sometimes is said that people "died from" given causes. However, according to the *American Medical Association Manual of Style* (Iverson et al. 1989, 145), the proper wording is "died of." Write that many people die of—not die from—strokes.

Eponyms

Many a title of a disease contains a person's name and thus is termed an eponym, which means "named after." Alzheimer's disease, Bright's disease, Cushing's disease, Down's syndrome . . . one can easily continue through the alphabet. As noted earlier, the person's name should be capitalized but not the rest of the disease name. Preference varies regarding whether to use the possessive form of the person's name—for example, whether to say "Parkinson's disease" or "Parkinson disease"; more and more publications seem to favor the latter. If in doubt, check with your editor about which form to use or, more broadly, which dictionary or style manual to consult.

Fever versus Temperature

Write that someone "had a temperature," and readers probably will understand what you mean. However, such wording is imprecise, as everyone has a temperature, be it high or low or in between. If someone's temperature was elevated, be precise: Write that the person had a fever. If relevant, indicate what the person's temperature was.

9.   Sensitivity and Style

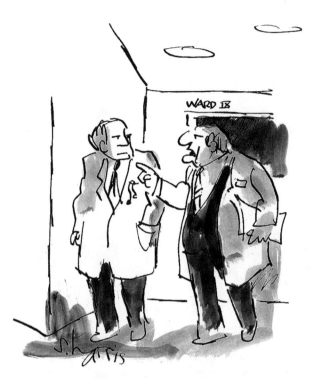

"REMEMBER THIS, RADKIN—I'VE GOT A DISEASE NAMED AFTER ME, AND YOU'VE ONLY GOT A SYNDROME."

Generic and Brand Names

Drugs that are commercially available typically have at least two names. Each drug has a generic, or nonproprietary, name—that is, the basic name of the drug, not protected by a trademark. In addition, drugs typically have one or more brand names, or trade names, supplied by their manufacturers. The drug with the generic name diazepam has the brand name Valium; that with the generic name diphenhydramine hydrochloride has the brand name Benadryl; and that with the generic name ibuprofen has the brand names Advil, Motrin, and Nuprin. Generic names of drugs are not capitalized, but brand names of drugs (like those of other products) are.

II. Preparing the Piece

In health writing, which of the two types of names should you use? The answer depends in part on the purpose of the writing. Often, for greatest clarity, both names should be mentioned early in a piece. In general, the generic name should be used thereafter, as the purpose is to inform the audience, not to promote a brand of drug. One exception is when a purpose is indeed to promote the brand—for example, in a publication by its manufacturer. Another is when distinguishing brands from each other is important—for example, if a problem has arisen with one brand of the drug.

Incidence and Prevalence

As discussed earlier, the terms "incidence" and "prevalence" are often confused. A reminder: "Incidence" refers to new cases, "prevalence" to existing cases. (To remember the difference, contrast the meanings of "inci-

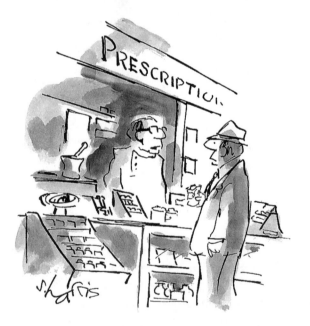

"THE GENERIC NAME FOR MEPLOSUTRICIN SNAKE-SKIN OIL."

dent" and "prevail.") The incidence rate is the number of new cases of a disease occurring in a population over a given period, divided by the size of the population. In contrast, the prevalence rate is the proportion of population members having the disease at a given time.

Life Expectancy versus Life Span

Also commonly confused are the terms "life expectancy" and "life span." Life span is the longest that members of a species can live; for example, humans have a greater life span than dogs. Life expectancy, in contrast, is how long—or how much longer—individuals under given circumstances are predicted, on average, to live. One can say that life expectancy at birth has increased in the last century; that cigarette smokers have a reduced life expectancy; or that people at a given stage of a certain disease have a typical life expectancy of two years.

Medicine and Physician

The terms "medicine" and "physician" can be ambiguous, for each has broad and narrow meanings. For example, virtually every school of medicine contains a department of medicine; yet clearly a single department is not the whole school. In the case of the school, "medicine" is meant broadly to include the entire field concerned with diagnosis, treatment, and prevention of disease. In the case of the department, however, "medicine" has its narrower meaning of internal medicine, the specialty concerned with nonsurgical care of adults.

"Physician" poses an analogous situation. In its broad sense, "physician" means simply medical doctor. In its narrow sense, however, "physician" means "internist"—that is, a medical doctor specializing in internal medicine. Thus, the American College of Physicians is an organization of internists, and the medical school at Columbia University is called the College of Physicians and Surgeons. Of course, "internist" should not be confused with "intern," a term sometimes used for a physician in the first year of residency training after graduation from medical school.

How to deal with these broad and narrow meanings? In your information-gathering, be clear in what sense these terms are being used. And of course be clear in your own writing, for example by saying "medical doctor" or "internist" if "physician" could be ambiguous.

II.   Preparing the Piece

Names of Institutions

A common error is to omit the final "s" from "Institutes" in the title "National Institutes of Health." NIH contains multiple institutes; hence the name is plural. Similarly, the correct name for CDC is the Centers (not Center) for Disease Control and Prevention. And if you write about, say, a medical exhibit at the Smithsonian, note that the correct name is the Smithsonian Institution, not the Smithsonian Institute.

In short, check that you have used the correct names for institutions you mention. Be aware that such names sometimes change; for instance, in earlier years CDC stood for Communicable Disease Center and then Center (singular) for Disease Control. Make sure that the designation you use is up to date.

Ophthalmologist, Optometrist, and Optician

An ophthalmologist (watch that spelling!) is a physician specializing in the eye; ophthalmologists do eye surgery as well as provide nonsurgical care. Optometrists, who have doctor of optometry degrees, are nonphysician health professionals providing mainly vision care. An optician is someone who makes and dispenses eyeglasses.

Psychiatrist and Psychologist

Another widespread error is to refer to "doctors and psychiatrists," as if psychiatrists were not doctors. Psychiatrists are indeed medical doctors: those who after medical school specialized in mental health and illness. To be accurate, "doctors and psychiatrists" should be changed to other wording, such as "doctors, including psychiatrists" or "psychiatrists and other doctors."

Also, psychiatrists and psychologists should not be confused with each other. Psychologists are specialists in the branch of science dealing with the mind and mental processes; commonly they have PhD degrees. Some psychologists work in clinical settings; others, however, focus solely on other pursuits, such as research and teaching.

Signs and Symptoms

When gathering information for health writing, you may come across references to "signs and symptoms." This phrase may seem redundant, for in everyday language "signs" and "symptoms" often mean the same thing. In medical language, however, a distinction exists: Signs are disease manifestations that can be objectively observed and often measured; examples include fever, swelling, and increased heart rate. Symptoms, however, are those manifestations subjectively experienced by the person with the disease—for instance, pain or itching or nausea.

In popular health writing, rarely will it be necessary to use the terms so precisely. Nevertheless, the distinction can be worth keeping in mind and the concept worth conveying. One reason: Even in this age of sophisticated diagnostic techniques, the history presented by the patient remains a prime source of information.

Traditionalism in Usage

Medical English, like other English, keeps evolving. Often, rules become less strict to accommodate common usage. For example, at one time a more definite distinction was drawn between "nauseous," which meant causing nausea, and "nauseated," which meant experiencing nausea. Today, however, in keeping with common usage, some authorities find it acceptable to use "nauseous" to mean experiencing nausea.

In health writing, it usually appears best to stick to more established usage. Doing so generally allows you to be more precise. It also helps keep you from annoying readers who follow traditional usage—and thus avoids distracting them from what you are saying. For some readerships, however, newer usage may be clearer and so should be followed. When in doubt, check recent dictionaries, consult your editor, define terms, and, as always, consider your audience.

Additional Items of Usage

As well as following proper medical usage, health writing must conform to good general usage. Here are some items of the latter that arise particularly often in health writing.

Affect and Effect

Health writing often deals with effects. In general, "effect" is the noun, "affect" the verb. For example, "The drug had a rapid effect on blood pressure" and "The drug affected blood pressure rapidly."

Some exceptions, however: "Affect" as a noun refers to the external expression of emotion. You may read, for instance, that a patient had a "flat affect." This technical wording should rarely be used in popular health writing. Also, "effect" as a verb means to cause, as in "The new medical director hopes to effect many changes."

Compare to and Compare with

Health writers often present comparisons. When entities of like category are being compared, "compare with" should be used. For example: "The results of the new operation were compared with those of the traditional one." The wording "compare to" should be used only when parallels are being drawn rather than actual comparisons made. Thus: "She compared the disease to a wolf" or "He compared his medical school professor to the near-legendary Sir William Osler."

Comprise

"Comprise" means encompass. Thus, one may correctly say, for example, "The clinic staff comprises doctors, nurses, and dietitians." It is incorrect to say that the staff "is comprised of" these three groups, just as it is incorrect to say that it "is encompassed of" them. Rather, one would say "composed of."

In general, "comprise" is best avoided. Even if you use it right, it often sounds wrong. "Consist of" or "composed of" can convey the needed meaning without the awkwardness of "comprise."

Continual and Continuous

"Continual" means repeated, "continuous" uninterrupted. For example, hiccuping that does not cease is continual. But pain that does not cease is continuous.

Criterion, Criteria; Phenomenon, Phenomena

"Criterion" and "phenomenon" are singular, "criteria" and "phenomena" plural. Thus "The main criterion was effectiveness of the treatment regimen; other criteria were cost and convenience." Or, "Yawning is a puzzling phenomenon. Phenomena that seem better understood include blinking, sneezing, and coughing."

9.   Sensitivity and Style

Different From

The correct wording is "different from," not "different than." (To remember this, think of "differs from.") For instance: "The curriculum at this dental school is different from that at most others."

Often, substituting "differs from" for "is different from" makes a sentence more concise: "The curriculum at this dental school differs from that at most others." Likewise, substituting "resembles" for "is similar to" can yield a crisper result.

Fewer versus Less

"Fewer" should be used for items that can be counted, "less" for those that cannot. For example: "People who had received the treatment missed fewer days of work and made fewer visits to the clinic. They also took less medication and reported less discomfort."

Follow up versus Follow-up

"Follow up" is a verb, "follow-up" a noun or adjective. Some examples: The researchers plan to follow up on these intriguing results. Careful follow-up is important in patients receiving this drug. This follow-up study will begin next month.

Gender-Neutral Wording

Health writing should, of course, use gender-neutral wording. Indeed, such wording is becoming so much the norm that examples of sexist wording are becoming difficult to find.

One aspect of using gender-neutral wording consists of avoiding sexist terms, such as "medical men" for "doctors." Another consists of avoiding irrelevant references to gender, as in "lady surgeon" or "male nurse." Another consists of not using "he" or "his" when reference to people of both genders is meant.

One approach to correcting the last problem is to convert the singular to the plural: Instead of saying "The biomedical researcher who works at a university must obtain grants to support his work," say "Biomedical researchers who work at universities must obtain grants to support their work." Another approach that sometimes works is to rephrase the sentence without a pronoun or to use the second person: Instead of "After he drafts a piece, the health writer should check all names and statistics," say

II.   Preparing the Piece

"After drafting a piece, the health writer should check all names and statistics" or "After drafting a piece, check all names and statistics."

Further guidance in writing gender-neutrally may be obtained from various books on the subject, such as *The Dictionary of Bias-Free Usage* (Maggio 1991) and *Guidelines for Bias-Free Writing* (Schwartz et al. 1995). Many writing textbooks and style manuals also offer guidance in this regard.

Hopefully

"Hopefully" means "in a hopeful manner," not "it is hoped." It is correct to say, "The patient thought hopefully about rehabilitation"—but incorrect to say, "Hopefully, a cure for this disease will be developed soon." To express the latter thought, sometimes an alternative to using such correct but awkward wording as "it is to be hoped" is to quote someone expressing the hope.

Nobel Prize

Health writing often refers to work that has won a Nobel Prize in physiology or medicine. Remember that the spelling is "Nobel" (after Alfred Nobel), not "Noble."

Sexual Orientation

Health writing often entails reference to sexual orientation. Preferred terminology has been changing, and different publications sometimes have different guidelines. If in doubt, consulting one's editor can be worthwhile.

It seems generally accepted, though, that the term "sexual orientation" should be used rather than "sexual preference." The former is more accurate, given that sexuality is rarely, if ever, simply a matter of choice. Also, in general the terms "lesbians" and "gay men" seem to be preferred for referring to these respective groups.

When referring to sexual orientation, beware of "heterosexism." For example, do not say that AIDS is an issue "not only for gay men but also for the general population." Everyone, regardless of sexual orientation or other characteristics, is part of the general population. A more accurate— and less marginalizing—wording would be "not only for gay men but also for the rest of the population."

Significant

In health writing, "significant" can mean either "important" or "large," or it can mean "statistically significant." (For a discussion of statistical significance, see Chapter 6.) In contexts where ambiguity may exist, avoid the word "significant." Rather, use a less ambiguous term or phrase.

That and Who

Use "who"—not "that"—to refer to people. For example, write "the physician assistant who performed the examination," not "the physician assistant that . . ."

Under Way

Health writers sometimes note that further studies are under way. Remember that when used as an adverb "under way" is two words, not one.

Unique

"Unique" means "one of a kind." Thus, something cannot be "fairly unique" or "very unique." In general, avoid the overused and often inaccurate word "unique." If a condition is rare or unusual, term it such; if a clinic has distinctive services, say that and explain what it distinctive about them. Do not be like the advertiser who said that "Many of our products are unique or even one of a kind."

To the beginning health writer, crafting material sensitively and following conventions of medical and general style may seem to entail undue effort. However, they are important to writing well about health. When you write, devote the time and thought that these items require. With experience, they will become almost automatic.

PART III

Exploring Areas and Issues

Chapter 10

(OVERING KEY REALMS

Heart disease, cancer, stroke. Infectious disease, mental illness, arthritis. Drugs, medical devices, surgical procedures. Health policy, the health care system, and more. Such is the stuff of health writing.

The current chapter provides some footholds for such key realms. It identifies institutional and other resources that can serve as starting points for gathering information. In some cases, it also provides guidance in presenting material obtained.

Information in this chapter complements that in earlier chapters that deal with techniques for gathering and presenting information. After gaining footholds from this chapter, consider returning to those sections for strategies that can aid you as you continue.

Diseases

A few diseases—or, more precisely, a few disease groups—account for most of the deaths in this country and for much of the illness. These diseases, their treatment, and their prevention can rightly receive considerable coverage. Here are some starting points for covering several such disease groups: heart disease, lung disease, cancer, infectious disease, neurologic disorders, mental illness, and arthritis. The material also can serve as a model for writing about diseases outside these groups.

Heart Disease

Diseases of the heart are the leading cause of death in the United States (Mortality Statistics Branch 1996). They are, therefore, the subject of much research. Efforts to prevent, diagnose, and treat them constitute a sizeable endeavor—and, indeed, a sizeable industry.

Here are some good starting points for information gathering on heart disease:

III. Exploring Areas and Issues

National Heart, Lung, and Blood Institute (NHLBI)
World Wide Web: http://www.nhlbi.nih.gov/nhlbi/nhlbi.htm
Phone: (301) 496-4236; (301) 251-1222 for information center
Comments: NHLBI is part of NIH.

American Heart Association (AHA)
World Wide Web: http://www.amhrt.org
Phone: (214) 706-1173 for media assistance; (800) 242-8721 toll-free for information; also see local phone directory
Fax: (214) 369-3685
Comments: See local phone directories for phone numbers of local AHA chapters.

Lung Disease

As its name indicates, the NHLBI also deals with lung disease, the fourth-leading cause of death. Another information source is the American Lung Association. Information from these institutions can be obtained as follows:

National Heart, Lung, and Blood Institute (NHLBI)
Comments: See listing above.

American Lung Association (ALA)
World Wide Web: http://www.lungusa.org
Phone: (212) 315-6473 for national media relations office; (800) LUNG-USA toll-free for local ALA offices
Fax: (212) 315-8872

Cancer

Basic information resources on cancer, the second most common cause of death in the United States can be found in the following sources:

National Cancer Institute (NCI)
World Wide Web: http://www.nci.nih.gov
Phone: (301) 496-6641 for mass media office; (800) 4-CANCER toll-free for cancer information service

Comments: NCI is part of NIH. It supplies cancer information by various means, including e-mail and fax.

American Cancer Society (ACS)
World Wide Web: http://www.cancer.org
Phone: (212) 382-2169 for national media office; (800) 227-2345 toll-free for information; also see local phone directory
Fax: (212) 719-0913

The Cancer Handbook: A Guide for the Nonspecialist
by Darrell E. Ward (Columbus: Ohio State University Press, 1995)
Comments: As well as explaining many cancer-related concepts and terms, this guide identifies sources from which to obtain information. Some of the basic-science material in this book can aid in covering research not only on cancer but also on other diseases.

What You Need to Know About Cancer
(special issue of *Scientific American*, September 1996)
Comments: Includes articles on the basic biology of cancer, causes and prevention, early detection, and therapy. Also includes briefings on 12 major cancers and a list of cancer information sources.

One thing to remember when writing about cancer is that it is a group of diseases. Prognosis varies considerably among types of cancer; it also can differ widely within a given type, depending in part on how early the disease was diagnosed and treated. Avoid the error of portraying cancer as a single disease for which the outlook is uniformly grim.

Infectious Disease

Once thought by some to be disappearing, infectious disease has again become an important problem for our society—and a major topic for health writers. Resources that can be good starting points are:

National Institute of Allergy and Infectious Diseases (NIAID)
World Wide Web: http://www.niaid.nih.gov
Phone: (301) 496-5717
Comments: NIAID is part of NIH.

III.   Exploring Areas and Issues

Centers for Disease Control and Prevention (CDC)
World Wide Web: http://www.cdc.gov
Phone: (404) 639-3286
Fax: (404) 639-7394
Comments: See Chapter 3 for additional material on CDC as an information source.

American Society for Microbiology (ASM)
World Wide Web: http://www.asmusa.org
Phone: (202) 942-9297
Fax: (202) 942-9367
E-Mail: communications@asmusa.org

Control of Communicable Diseases Manual, 16th ed.
by Abram S. Benenson (Washington, DC: American Public Health Association, 1995)
Comments: For each of more than 100 diseases ranging from acquired immunodeficiency syndrome to zygomycosis, this standard manual offers information on aspects such as infectious agent, diagnosis, mode of transmission, and control. The manual is updated periodically; look for the latest edition.

A Field Guide to Germs
by Wayne Biddle (New York: Henry Holt and Company, 1995)
Comments: This popularly oriented guide may be especially useful as a source of historical background.

Federal sources of information specifically on AIDS include the National AIDS Hotline, at telephone number (800) 342-AIDS, and the National AIDS Clearinghouse, at telephone number (800) 458-5231. In addition, the National Library of Medicine has published a guide to information services on AIDS and HIV that are available at NIH and selected other government sites (National Library of Medicine 1995).

Associations concerned with specific infectious diseases can be worth consulting. Of course, in interpreting materials from disease-related associations, one should remember that some groups are strongly involved in advocacy for people with the disease.

Medical writer Laurie Garrett, who has written extensively about infec-

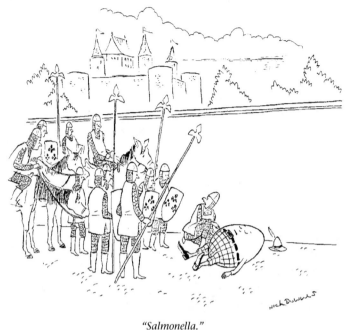

"Salmonella."

© 1989 by Nick Downes; from *Science.*

tious disease, offers the following advice for covering disease outbreaks (Garrett 1997): Take the time to learn about the microorganisms involved. Get to know public health officers beforehand rather than suddenly contacting them during a time of crisis; also develop sources at schools of medicine and public health. In settings where you are at risk of contracting the infection, take the same precautions as the scientists are taking. Further perspective is available in the chapter from which these points were taken.

Neurologic Disorders

Disorders of the nervous system cause much disability and many deaths—indeed, stroke is the third most common cause of death in the United States. Also, neuroscience is a highly active field of research. Both factors make neurology and neuroscience a major area for health writing. Resources that can be useful starting points include:

III. Exploring Areas and Issues

National Institute of Neurological Disorders and Stroke (NINDS)

World Wide Web: http://www.ninds.nih.gov

Phone: (301) 496-5924

Comments: NINDS is part of NIH. One NINDS publication that can especially aid health writers is the guide *Neurological Disorders: Voluntary Health Agencies and Other Patient Resources* (National Institute of Neurological Disorders and Stroke 1994), which lists and briefly describes organizations concerned with various conditions.

National Stroke Association (NSA)

World Wide Web: http://www.stroke.org

Phone: (303) 649-9299; (800)-STROKES toll-free for information

Fax: (303) 649-1328

Comments: The NSA has produced a reporter's handbook, *The Stroke/Brain Attack Reporter's Handbook,* (National Stroke Association 1995), that includes background information. Of course, any such handbook should be supplemented by sources that can be more current.

American Heart Association (AHA)

Phone: (800) 553-6321 toll-free for information on stroke

Comments: For information on the AHA, see listing under "Heart Disease" above.

Society for Neuroscience

World Wide Web: http://www.sfn.org

Phone: (202) 462-6688

Comments: The Society for Neuroscience focuses largely on neuroscience research. Its publication *Brain Facts: A Primer on the Brain and Nervous System* (Society for Neuroscience 1993) can provide good background.

Mental Illness

An area overlapping neuroscience is that of mental health and illness. About one person in five, it is estimated, experiences such illness in any given year (American Psychiatric Association 1994b). Initial resources to consult are:

National Institute of Mental Health (NIMH)

World Wide Web: http://www.nimh.nih.gov
Phone: (301) 443-4536
Fax: (301) 443-0008
E-Mail: nimhpress@nih.gov
Comments: NIMH is part of NIH.

American Psychiatric Association

World Wide Web: http://www.psych.org
Phone: (202) 682-6142
Fax: (202) 682-6255
E-Mail: paffairs@psych.org
Comments: The American Psychiatric Association has published a media guide, *Mental Illnesses Awareness Guide for the Media* (American Psychiatric Association 1994b), that includes background information on mental illnesses, a glossary, and a resource list.

American Psychological Association

World Wide Web: http://www.apa.org
Phone: (202) 336-5700
E-Mail: public.affairs@apa.org

National Mental Health Association (NMHA)

World Wide Web: http://www.nmha.org
Phone: (703) 684-7722; (800) 969-NMHA toll-free for information
Fax: (703) 684-5968

Diagnostic and Statistical Manual of Mental Disorders, 4th ed.

(Washington, DC: American Psychiatric Association, 1994)
Comments: Standard reference work describing mental disorders. Commonly known as DSM-IV.

Stories on mental illnesses, like those on other conditions, often benefit from human interest. However, special issues can arise in interviewing and writing about the people affected. For example, some people with mental illnesses can have particular difficulty grasping the implications of being interviewed; thus, they can be vulnerable to exploitation. Given certain social attitudes, publishing some types of information can be hurtful to the people portrayed or those around them. Awareness of such issues can aid in approaching this area sensitively, as can consultation of institutional sources such as those noted above. For a case study and some guidelines, see the article "Sarah's Story" by journalist Cathryn Creno (1992).

Arthritis

Nearly 40 million Americans of all ages have some type of arthritis (Arthritis Foundation n.d.), which literally means inflammation of a joint or joints. And as the population becomes older, the number is expected to increase. Basic resources regarding arthritis include:

National Institute of Arthritis and Musculoskeletal and Skin Diseases (NIAMS)
World Wide Web: http://www.nih.gov/niams
Phone: (301) 496-8188; (301) 495-4484 for clearinghouse
Comments: NIAMS is part of NIH.

Arthritis Foundation
World Wide Web: http://www.arthritis.org
Phone: (404) 872-7100; (800) 283-7800 toll-free for information; also see local phone directory
Fax: (404) 872-0457
Comments: The Arthritis Foundation has prepared *The Arthritis Fact Book for the Media* (Arthritis Foundation n.d).

Organizations focusing on specific types of arthritis also exist. They can be identified through the sources noted above, as well as through online and printed directories such as those listed in Chapter 3.

Health writers should keep in mind that arthritis is not a single disease. Rather, the term refers to more than 100 conditions affecting the joints. Care should be taken to avoid the easy trap of confusing one type of arthritis with another, such as rheumatoid arthritis with osteoarthritis.

Health-Care Technologies

Much health writing deals with health-care technologies—the means of preventing, diagnosing, and treating disease. Such technologies include, but are not limited to, drugs, medical devices, and surgical operations. They encompass approaches in both mainstream and alternative medicine.

Mainstream Medical Technologies

Many resources are available for covering technologies in mainstream medicine. Some good basic starting points are:

Food and Drug Administration (FDA)
World Wide Web: http://www.fda.gov
Phone: (301) 827-6242
Comment: The FDA's responsibilities include regulating drugs and medical devices in the United States.

Office of Medical Applications of Research (OMAR)
World Wide Web: http://text.nlm.nih.gov/nih/uploadv3/
About/OMAR/OMAR.html
Phone: (301) 496-1144
Comment: OMAR is part of NIH. Its activities include holding "consensus conferences" to evaluate biomedical technologies. The resulting consensus statements, as well as other NIH technology assessment statements, are available through the OMAR Web site. They also can be ordered from the NIH Consensus Program Information Center, toll-free telephone (888) 644-2667.

National Library of Medicine, Health Services/Technology
World Wide Web: http://text.nlm.nih.gov/ftrs-v3/gateway
Comments: Items available through this site include Agency for Health Care Policy and Research guidelines, which include recommendations for management of various medical conditions.

ECRI
World Wide Web: http://www.hslc.org/emb
Phone: (610) 825-6000
Fax: (610) 834-1275
E-Mail: ecri@hslc.org
Comment: ECRI, a nonprofit agency, evaluates medical devices and other health technologies and then publishes reports. It has been com-

pared to Consumers Union, publisher of *Consumer Reports* (Stephenson 1995).

Of course, manufacturers and the groups that represent them also can serve as sources. The organization Pharmaceutical Research and Manufacturers of America (PhRMA) can be contacted at telephone number (202) 835-3400, and the Health Industry Manufacturers Association (HIMA) can be reached at (202) 783-8700. Each year PhRMA issues a reporter's handbook (PhRMA 1996) that includes telephone numbers of media contacts at pharmaceutical companies and selected other health-related institutions.

The *Physicians' Desk Reference* (1997) is a standard reference work on drugs. And the book *Introduction to Reference Sources in the Health Sciences* (Roper and Boorkman 1994) contains a chapter, "Drug Information Sources" (Fishman 1994), identifying many sources of drug information.

Recently an ongoing initiative was begun to review the evidence available from clinical trials of various medical interventions. This large international initiative, known as the Cochrane Collaboration (Bero and Rennie 1995, Taubes 1996b), is yielding a collection of continually updated reports. The Cochrane Collaboration home page can be accessed at http://hiru.mcmaster.ca/cochrane/default.htm. Information may also be obtained from the U.S. Cochrane Information Clearinghouse, telephone (210) 617-5190.

In writing about health care technologies, remember to keep the big picture in mind. As well as dealing with a given technology, compare it with alternatives, and consider not only benefits but also risks and costs. Explore also whether the technology poses ethical issues. In short, provide the context needed to put your subject in perspective.

Alternative Medicine

Complementary and alternative medicine—which the NIH defines as "those practices used for the prevention and treatment of disease that are not taught widely in medical schools, nor generally available inside hospitals"—is gaining considerable attention in the United States. Examples of the many systems or approaches commonly viewed as complementary or alternative include homeopathy, osteopathy, chiropractic, herbalism, aromatherapy, traditional Chinese medicine, Ayurveda, and Native American medicine. In a study reported in the *New England Journal of Medicine*, about one in three Americans who were surveyed reported using at least one unconventional therapy in the past year (Eisenberg et al. 1993).

Alternative medicine seems to be a growing focus for health writing. It is also increasingly becoming a perspective to include in general coverage of health-related topics. Basic resources that may be useful to consult:

Office of Alternative Medicine (OAM)
Phone: (301) 496-1712; (888) 644-6226 toll-free for OAM Clearinghouse
Fax: (301) 480-7660
Comments: OAM, a part of NIH, was created in 1992. Its purpose is to "facilitate the evaluation of alternative medical treatment modalities" and to help integrate effective such treatments into mainstream medical practice.

The Alternative Medicine Homepage
http://www.pitt.edu/~cbw/altm.html

Alternative Medicine: Expanding Medical Horizons
(Washington, DC: U.S. Government Printing Office, 1994)
Comments: Subtitled "A Report to the National Institutes of Health on Alternative Medical Systems and Practices in the United States." Describes fields of practice and discusses conducting and disseminating research.

Fundamentals of Complementary and Alternative Medicine
edited by Marc S. Micozzi (New York: Churchill Livingstone, 1996)
Comments: Provides general background on complementary and alternative medicine as well as discussing various systems and approaches. Contains many references.

Alternative Therapies in Health and Medicine
Comments: This is a peer-reviewed journal, recently established.

In writing about alternative medicine, as in other health writing, balance seems to be the key. Approach your task with an open mind, but critically evaluate what you learn. Say what is known and what isn't, and differentiate evidence from opinion. Present your material with sensitivity and respect but also with professional impartiality. Then your writing about alternative medicine can truly complement that about more conventional medical technologies.

III.   Exploring Areas and Issues

Health Policy, Health Care, and Related Areas

Contexts for considering health-care technologies often include health policy and the health-care system. These areas are in themselves major areas for health writing.

Abigail Trafford, health editor of the *Washington Post*, has written a helpful chapter titled "Critical Coverage of Public Health and Government" (Trafford 1997). Trafford emphasizes the importance of consulting a variety of sources when covering government health policies and programs. In addition to government officials, she states, these sources should include experts at major institutions (schools of public health, hospital systems, and policy centers, for example), representatives of advocacy and lobby groups (such as disease organizations and health-related trade associations), people directly affected by the health problem, and the general public. Trafford also notes the need to be aware of political spin, and the importance of considering who stands to gain or lose financially from given policies or programs.

Guidance in covering the health care system is available in "Focus on Healthcare: A Handbook for Journalists" (Lieberman 1993), published as a special section of the *Columbia Journalism Review*. This journalists' handbook on health care contains a substantial glossary of terms regarding the health-care system. It also lists many organizations of various types that can serve as sources. Although this handbook is somewhat dated, it can be a good starting point. More recently, the *Columbia Journalism Review* published a brief but substantive list of resources, "The Next Round of Health Care Hotspots" (Gentry 1995), for reporting on health maintenance organizations (HMOs).

Sources of guidance for investigative reporting on health care include the organization Investigative Reporters and Editors (IRE). For information on IRE and resources available from it, see Chapter 8.

Other Realms

Two other major areas for health writing are aging and injury prevention.

Aging

As older people constitute more and more of the population, aging is becoming an increasingly important topic for health writers. Basic resources in this realm include:

148

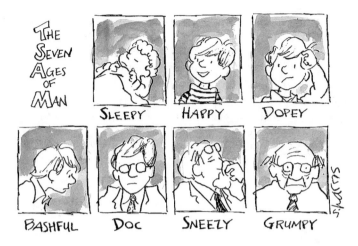

THE SEVEN AGES OF MAN

SLEEPY   HAPPY   DOPEY

BASHFUL   DOC   SNEEZY   GRUMPY

© Sidney Harris, reproduced by permission.

National Institute on Aging (NIA)
World Wide Web: http://www.nih.gov/nia
Phone: (301) 496-1752; (800) 222-2225 for NIA information center
Comments: NIA is part of NIH.

American Geriatrics Society
World Wide Web: http://www.americangeriatrics.org
Phone: (212) 308-1414, (800) 247-4779 (toll-free)
Fax: (212) 832-8646
E-Mail: info.amger@amgeriatrics.org
Comments: The American Geriatrics Society has produced a popularly oriented book on aging and health, *The American Geriatrics Society's Complete Guide to Aging and Health* (Williams 1995), that can be a good source of background.

Gerontological Society of America
World Wide Web: http://www.geron.org
Phone: (202) 842-1275
Fax: (202) 842-1150
Comments: The Gerontological Society has a large pool of experts to recommend for interviews.

III.   Exploring Areas and Issues

Injury Prevention

Unintentional injuries are the fifth-leading cause of death in the United States. Often affecting the young or middle-aged, they are the leading cause of years of potential life lost before age 65 (National Safety Council 1995). Some basic resources on this subject are:

National Safety Council
World Wide Web: http://www.nsc.org
Phone: (630) 285-1121, (800) 621-7619 (toll-free)
Fax: (630) 285-1315
Comments: The National Safety Council produces the annual publication *Accident Facts* (National Safety Council 1996), which contains statistics on unintentional injuries.

Centers for Disease Control and Prevention
Comments: See listing above (under "Infectious Disease"). The CDC includes the National Center for Injury Prevention and Control.

The Injury Fact Book, 2d ed.
by Susan P. Baker et al. (New York: Oxford University Press, 1992)
Comments: Provides statistics and other information.

As you may notice as you gather information, the public health community generally prefers to speak of "unintentional injuries" rather than "accidents." The rationale: Whereas "accident" implies an uncontrollable act of fate, "injury" does not and thus is more compatible with promoting prevention. In writing for the public, the term "accident" may sometimes be clearer and more efficient. But whatever wording is chosen, prevention should be emphasized.

This chapter has touched on some of the key realms that health writers cover. May the content help you gain footholds when you approach topics in these realms. And may it serve as a model for approaching topics in other realms as well.

Chapter 11

PRESENTING RISK

Risks posed by environmental hazards. Risks associated with behaviors or lack thereof. Risks stemming from genetic factors. Risks presented by medical treatments. Whether working for the media or in institutional settings, health writers often communicate about known or postulated risks.

Though risk is a short and simple and common word, it can be a tricky concept to communicate. Fortunately, researchers have been exploring how people tend to perceive risk and accordingly how to present it. Although much of this work comes from the field of environmental communication, many of the findings and recommendations also seem applicable to communicating about health risks other than those posed by environmental factors.

Drawing on overviews of this work (Castelli 1990; Kamrin, Katz, and Walter 1995; Oleckno 1995; West, Sandman, and Greenberg 1995), this chapter begins by discussing how members of the public tend to perceive risk. It then offers pointers on risk presentation. Finally, it identifies some resources to use in writing about environmental risks.

Understanding Risk Perception

To the scientific community, risk is mainly a statistical concept: the likelihood that in given circumstances a given unfavorable event will occur. However, the public's view of a risk entails more than numbers.

People typically view the natural as safer and more acceptable than the artificial. For example, foods tend to be seen as safe, but food additives as dangerous, even when evidence exists to the contrary; likewise, the risks of contraception evoke more concern than the greater risks of pregnancy. The familiar usually is seen as safer than the unfamiliar; a home tends to seem less dangerous than a factory, even when it is not. And risks posed by chronic factors, such as lifestyle, tend to be underestimated relative to those of sudden, catastrophic events.

The nature of the outcome also influences risk perception. Items causing dread diseases evoke more concern than those producing diseases that are equally serious but less feared. For instance, an agent causing deaths from cancer tends to seem more risky than one causing as many deaths from heart disease, asthma, or diabetes. Furthermore, the risk of items that cause catastrophic or memorable outcomes tends to be magnified in people's minds. Because plane crashes kill many people at once and receive much media attention, plane travel tends to seem more dangerous than it is.

Context likewise affects views of risk. Risks from voluntary behaviors—such as tobacco or alcohol use, or dangerous sports—seem less weighty than risks that are involuntary, such as those from a nearby factory's wastes. Similarly, risks subject to one's own control loom smaller than those over which one has little or no control. And risks that are unfair—with benefits and risks accruing to different people—tend to be perceived as particularly serious. Thus, treatments posing high risks may be acceptable to patients with otherwise fatal diseases, but even a low risk from industrial pollution may be alarming to a community that feels it gains little from the industry. In keeping with the example of the treatment, risks tend to be seen as more acceptable if no reasonable alternative exists.

Risks tend to be more frightening, and thus viewed as more grave, if uncertainty about their magnitude exists or if the agent of risk is not readily detectable. In addition, the seriousness assigned to a risk depends in part on the credibility of the person or group presenting the information. For example, risk information from a trusted physician may be interpreted differently from that given by a representative of a drug company or factory.

One way that some environmental-communication experts distinguish the narrow statistical sense of risk from its broader, more complex perception is to invoke the concept of outrage. Hazards that engender outrage—because they are unfair or otherwise repugnant—are perceived as greater, or more worthy of concern than those hazards that are somehow accepted as parts of normal life. By keeping in mind this emotional aspect of risk perception, health writers can more effectively present information and guidance regarding risks.

Presenting Risk

So, how to go about presenting risk? Here are 10 suggestions that draw both on observations above and on material in earlier chapters.

11. Presenting Risk

(1) Consider carefully which risks to write about: Often the hazards that at first seem most newsworthy—those associated with disasters or caused by environmental disruption rather than lifestyle factors—are not those with greatest impact on health. When evaluating story ideas relating to risk, consider such aspects as the size of the risk and the amenability of the risk factor to control. Think accordingly how much of a story, if any, the subject merits. Because attention in the media can help brand a risk as important, being a responsible health writer requires such a thoughtful approach.

(2) Indicate the nature, source, and consistency of the evidence: Does evidence of risk come from animal studies? epidemiologic research? other investigation? Were the findings presented in a peer-reviewed journal? at a conference? elsewhere? Was the work funded by government? industry? another source? Has more than one study been done? If so, how consistent are the findings, and what range of estimates has emerged? What are the limitations of the research thus far? What remains unknown? Seek answers to such questions and present the answers when you write about risk.

(3) Distinguish facts from opinions: Given the uncertainty that commonly exists, statements about risk often reflect expert (or not-so-expert) opinion rather than evidence. Find out which statements are supported by findings and which ones venture beyond them. Clearly distinguish the two in your writing.

(4) Present absolute as well as relative risks: Saying merely that a given exposure doubles the likelihood of developing a given condition does not convey much useful information. As illustrated in Chapter 6, depending on whether the condition is rare or common, the impact could vary widely. Thus, in addition to stating relative risks, be sure to provide information on the absolute magnitude of the effect—for example, the number of people affected.

(5) Consider framing risks in more than one way (Castelli 1990): To communicate most fully, consider presenting statistics on risk from more than one standpoint. Saying that 1 person in 100 experiences a given effect may convey one impression; saying that 99 people in 100 do not may convey another. Presenting the information both ways may allow the audience to grasp the situation better.

(6) Consider comparing one risk with others: Providing comparisons can help the audience put a risk in perspective. Take care, however, only to make comparisons that are valid. Beware of comparing the risk posed by an involuntary exposure, such as that to a pollutant, with that presented by a voluntary action. In comparing risks, it sometimes is helpful to show a range—for example, to present the likelihood of injury from a given item on a spectrum including both safer and more hazardous items.

(7) Put risks in the context of benefits: Making decisions about health often entails weighing risks against benefits. Remember to present information

III. Exploring Areas and Issues

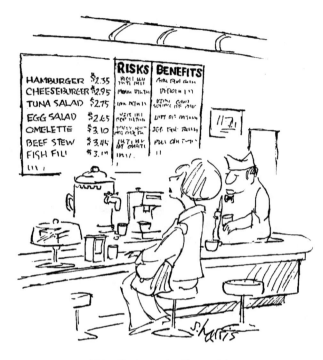

© Sidney Harris, reproduced by permission.

on both. For instance, when reporting on dangers of a medical interven-
tion, also identify the nature and likelihood of benefits. If relevant, present risks and benefits in the context of monetary and other costs.

(8) Discuss alternatives: Many conditions in medicine can be prevented, diagnosed, or treated in more than one way. Likewise, different public-health
actions can achieve similar effects. And industry can sometimes accomplish a goal through various means. Thus, rather than considering the
risks of a given technology or policy or process in isolation, compare them
with those of alternative approaches.

(9) Discuss measures for controlling risk: If risks are ones that institutions
such as industry or government can reduce, indicate what is—and is not—
being done. When relevant, let people know how they can spur such institutions to do more. Empower people by telling them what they can do to
reduce their own risk.

(10) Consider how to counter unrealistic perceptions: As noted earlier, people's
perceptions of the seriousness of a risk sometimes are inconsistent with
the size of the risk. These perceptions can make sense from a psychological
standpoint, but they can lead people to ignore major risks to health while
devoting great attention to those posing little danger. Therefore these per-

ceptions are sometimes worth countering. One approach for doing so is that proposed by Rowan (1990) for "transformative explanations." As discussed in Chapter 7, this approach entails stating the common view and acknowledging its plausibility before showing the greater adequacy of the scientifically founded view. Understanding factors affecting risk perception can aid in noting why the common view is plausible. And the respectfulness of this approach may avoid adding to outrage and thus aid in persuasion.

Covering Environmental Risk: Some Resources

Health writers as well as environmental writers may cover environmental risks. Some basic resources for doing so are identified below.

Environmental Protection Agency (EPA)
World Wide Web: http://www.epa.gov
Phone: (202) 260-7963; (202) 260-5922 for public information center

National Institute of Environmental Health Sciences (NIEHS)
World Wide Web: http://www.niehs.nih.gov
Phone: (919) 541-3345
Comments: NIEHS is part of NIH.

Occupational Safety and Health Administration (OSHA)
World Wide Web: http://www.osha.gov
Phone: (202) 219-8151

Centers for Disease Control and Prevention (CDC)
Comments: CDC includes the National Center for Environmental Health and the National Institute for Occupational Safety and Health. For guidance in obtaining information from CDC, see Chapters 3 and 10.

Toxicology and Environmental Health Information Program (TEHIP)
World Wide Web: http://sis.nlm.nih.gov/tehip1.htm
Phone: (301) 496-1131
Fax: (301) 480-3537
E-Mail: tehip@teh.nlm.nih.gov

III. Exploring Areas and Issues

Comments: TEHIP is a National Library of Medicine program offering on-line access to various information resources, including the databases in the Toxicology Data Network (TOXNET). The program also responds to queries.

Society of Environmental Journalists (SEJ)
Comments: The SEJ home page, at http://www.sej.org, offers access to many other Web sites relating to the environment. For guidance in contacting SEJ, see Chapter 14.

The Reporter's Environmental Handbook
by Bernadette West, Peter M. Sandman, and Michael R. Greenberg (New Brunswick, NJ: Rutgers University Press, 1995)
Comments: This book consists largely of chapters on various environmental risks; as well as summarizing knowledge about the risks, the chapters discuss measures for their control, sources useful in reporting on them, and pitfalls for writers to avoid. Chapters likely to interest health writers include those on asbestos, birth defects, cancer cluster claims, and occupational exposure to toxic chemicals. The book also discusses risk communication.

Reporting on Risk: A Journalist's Handbook on Environmental Risk Assessment
by Michael A. Kamrin, Dolores J. Katz, and Martha L. Walter (Los Angeles: Foundation for American Communications, 1995)
Comments: Major areas addressed include basics of assessing risk, exposure, and toxicity. The book also discusses risk communication.

Improving Risk Communication
by the Committee on Risk Perception and Communication (Washington, DC: National Academy Press, 1989)
Comments: This report, issued by the National Research Council, remains a useful resource.

"Toxics and Risk Reporting"
by Richard Harris, in *A Field Guide for Science Writers,* edited by Deborah Blum and Mary Knudson (New York: Oxford University Press, 1997)
Comments: A useful brief discussion by a leading science reporter.

11.   Presenting Risk

Even for the expert health writer, presenting risk can pose difficult challenges. However, by understanding risk perception, following basic guidelines, and drawing on suitable resources, you can succeed in this important task. Given the importance of the information you may be conveying, the effort can be most worthwhile.

Chapter 12

ETHICAL ISSUES

In a sense, this entire book is about ethics, for it deals with being a responsible health writer. Choosing topics soundly, researching them well, evaluating information rigorously, and presenting it effectively and sensitively all are parts of being a health writer who is not only good in a technical sense but also in a moral sense. So are pursuing a worthwhile career path and keeping oneself well educated, the topics of the remaining section of this book.

Some of these areas, however, pose particular ethical issues, and some ethical concerns in health writing overlap or fall outside the areas discussed. Thus, this chapter focuses on ethical issues that health writers face. The chapter begins by briefly discussing approaches to such issues. Then it presents codes of ethics developed by two health writers' organizations. Finally, the chapter addresses some major areas in which ethical issues tend to arise in health writing: choice of topics and content, choice of employers and publication sites, conflict of interest, privacy and confidentiality, depiction of disfigurement and dysfunction, use of media to garner resources, and participation in writing contests.

This chapter provides few answers, for by definition ethical dilemmas entail weighing competing values. It is hoped, however, that the chapter will raise awareness of the types of ethical issues health writers face so that such issues can be recognized more fully and dealt with more explicitly. It is also hoped that material in this chapter may serve as a model for approaching situations not discussed.

Approaches to Ethical Issues in Health Writing

When ethical issues arise in health writing—for example, whether to pursue a given topic or include a given piece of information—various questions can be worth considering. What good is likely to result from the action? What harm could result? Is the action consistent with such basic values as truthfulness? Is the action fair—or does it favor some people over others? Is the action consistent with a respectful and caring approach to other people? Are there alternatives to consider?

III.   Exploring Areas and Issues

Discussing such questions with others can be useful. Editors often can provide useful perspective; and indeed, when some types of ethical issues arise, it is the writer's responsibility to talk with the editor. Fellow writers also can be of help; consider consulting those with whom you work or those with similar positions to yours at other publications or institutions. If you know an ethicist who is attuned to the world of health writing, perhaps consult such a person as well.

In addition, you can draw on written resources. Articles on ethical issues in health writing continually appear; try keeping a file of readings and updating it periodically. Among possible items to include are the entry "Media and Medicine" (Elliott 1995) in the *Encyclopedia of Bioethics,* the health-related articles (Baggot 1992, Cohn 1992, Schwitzer 1992, Steele 1992) from a special ethics section that appeared in the journalism magazine *Quill,* and other articles cited in this chapter. Additional written resources include health writers' codes of ethics, the topic of the section below.

Codes of Ethics

Both the American Medical Writers Association (AMWA) and the National Association of Physician Broadcasters (NAPB) have issued codes of ethics. The codes are reprinted as figures 12-1 and 12-2.

These codes differ somewhat in scope, reflecting the different compositions of the organizations. For example, the AMWA code includes material on observing statutes and regulations, as many AMWA members work for the pharmaceutical and medical-device industries and thus must comply with rules of the Food and Drug Administration. The NAPB code mentions avoiding journalistic exploitation of one's patients, a concern when journalists also are clinicians.

The two codes, however, have some major aspects in common. For example, both emphasize accurate, balanced, well-informed reporting. Also, both call for respecting confidentiality.

Before proceeding further in this chapter, you are encouraged to read the AMWA and NAPB codes. Especially in the latter, you will find echoes of various points made earlier in this book. And Principle 5 in the former, which calls for continuing education, helps set the stage for coming chapters. As you read the codes, consider which points apply most to the type of work you are doing or plan to do. And given that ethics can contain areas of controversy, consider why you agree or disagree with various points.

Figure 12-1:   American Medical Writers Association Code of Ethics

Preamble
The American Medical Writers Association (AMWA) is an educational organization that promotes advances and challenges in biomedical communications by recommending principles of conduct for its members. These principles take into account the important role of biomedical communicators in writing, editing, and developing materials in various media and the potential of the products of their efforts to inform, educate, and influence audiences. To uphold the dignity and honor of their profession and of AMWA, biomedical communicators should accept the ethical principles and engage only in activities that bring credit to their profession, to AMWA, and to themselves.

Principle 1
Biomedical communicators should recognize and observe statutes and regulations pertaining to the materials they write, edit, or otherwise develop.

Principle 2
Biomedical communicators should apply objectivity, scientific accuracy and rigor, and fair balance while conveying pertinent information in all media.

Principle 3
Biomedical communicators should write, edit, or participate in the development of information that meets the highest professional standards, whether or not such materials come under the purview of any regulatory agency. They should attempt to prevent the perpetuation of incorrect information.
    Biomedical communicators should accept an assignment only when working in collaboration with a qualified specialist in the area, or when they are adequately prepared to undertake the assignment by training, experience, or ongoing study.

Principle 4
Biomedical communicators should work only under conditions or terms that allow proper application of their judgment and skills. They should refuse to participate in assignments that require unethical or questionable practices.

Principle 5
Biomedical communicators should expand and perfect their professional knowledge and communications skills.

Principle 6
Biomedical communicators should respect the confidential nature of materials provided to them. They should not divulge, without appropriate permission, any confidential patent, proprietary, or patient information.

Figure 12-1: *(continued)*

Principle 7
Biomedical communicators should expect and accept fair and reasonable remuneration and acknowledgment for their services. They should honor the terms of any contract or agreements into which they enter.

Principle 8
Biomedical communicators should consider their membership in AMWA an honor and a trust. They should conduct themselves accordingly in their professional interactions.

Original: Eric W. Martin, Ph.D., 1973
First revision: June 1989
Second revision: April 1994

Figure 12-2: National Association of Physician Broadcasters Code of Ethics

---

The National Association of Physician Broadcasters, as the official organization of physicians in print and electronic media, endorses a standard of behavior based on the tenets and traditions of the professions of Medicine and Journalism. Mass communication has a direct impact on the health and welfare of the American people. As agents of that communication, we recognize public enlightenment as the foundation of personal freedom and independence and we acknowledge a responsibility to perform within the following standards of practice:

I. ACCURACY: We believe our highest responsibility is to provide clear, concise, current, and accurate health information to the American public in support of participatory health care.
  1. Information provided should always be truthful and well substantiated.
  2. Sources of information should be fully disclosed.
  3. We should never extend beyond the boundaries of our knowledge base.
  4. Areas of medical doubt or controversy should be clearly defined and communicated.
  5. Where appropriate, conflicting points of view should be represented.

II. INDEPENDENCE: In the pursuit of accuracy and truth, we recognize the need to function in a fully credible and independent manner.
  1. We affirm the constitutional right of freedom of the press and the principle of the public's right to know.
  2. Gifts or special privileges that would compromise personal independence and integrity should not be accepted.

Figure 12-2: *(continued)*

3. Participation in organizations that would compromise personal objectivity should be avoided.
4. Editorial comments and other statements of opinion should be clearly labeled as such.
5. All sources of funding to develop content or secure access to print or electronic media should be fully disclosed with content presentation.

III. PERSONAL RIGHTS: We acknowledge and support the unalienable rights of people in a free society and our responsibility to support those rights.
1. We acknowledge the right of people to question and challenge actions and ideas of individuals and organizations.
2. We acknowledge the right of each individual to privacy, dignity, and confidentiality.
3. We acknowledge that people and institutions are innocent until proven guilty.
4. We acknowledge a special responsibility to protect our personal patients from any practice that might be viewed as exploitative.
5. We acknowledge the right of our audience, as extensions of our own patients, to a standard of interaction that is respectful, courteous, and consistent with the teachings of the profession of Medicine.

IV. CONTINUITY: Dedication to patient involvement in health care, a family centered emphasis, and support of social activism based in sound public health policy are central to our mission and reflect a commitment to strong continuity of care.
1. Providing diagnoses and treatments in the absence of physician examination and consultation is to be avoided.
2. General therapeutic advice, in areas supported by an adequate knowledge base, when provided to support healthful behaviors or encourage further evaluation, is appropriate.
3. Thorough definition of the risks versus gains of differing modalities of care is essential.
4. Complete delineation of the possible repercussions of various approaches to care, including the avoidance of care, should be well defined.
5. Clear definition of the importance of face-to-face evaluations with health care providers and proper follow-up should be reinforced.

V. CONTENT: As physicians and journalists, we accept the responsibility to distribute information that will best serve the needs of the American public.
1. Content selection should be based on its potential positive impact on health.
2. Content selection based on sensationalism or ratings appeal unaccompanied by redeemable positive health impact should be avoided.
3. Evaluation of the cost and quality of health care should be integral to the content development process.

Figure 12-2: *(continued)*

4. Emphasis should be placed on educational and instructional design with clearly defined health missions.
5. Whenever possible, activities should be linked to existing community health resources, in the hopes that such networking might enhance the program's beneficial effects.
   Adopted 1991.

Reprinted by permission.

Areas Posing Ethical Issues

Whatever the setting in which you work, various ethical issues can arise as you write about health. Health writers for the popular media, those in public information offices of institutions, and those doing freelance work face many of the same issues. They also face issues distinctive to their settings. Presented below are some of the main issues that health writers face. They are discussed in the context of questions and codes presented earlier in this chapter.

Choice of Topics and Content

Ethical issues begin with the very choice of what to write about. A health writer, one might claim, should write that which will do good. Given a choice of topics, it follows that the health writer should pursue that which will do most good.

Would that it were so easy. The impact of health writing can be difficult to predict. And further, what does it mean for health writing to do *good?* Does health writing do good only if it helps people improve their health or stay well? What if it contributes to bettering medical care? What if it increases people's basic medical knowledge or helps people learn to assess medical information? What about health writing that allays needless worries? Or health writing that addresses matters important to some people's quality of life? For instance, is writing about cosmetic surgery a valid use of a health writer's skill? What about writing that helps the community understand and accept people with disabilities or diseases? What about writing that engenders support for medical research? Or writing that helps a medical institution or organization thrive and thus allows it to contribute more to health? And given that the intellectual and the aesthetic and the entertaining can be considered goods in themselves, what about health writing that mainly enlightens or appeals or delights?

Different health writers have different answers to such questions. And different health writers, having different values, rank goals of health writing differently. No one set of right answers exists. Indeed, the same health writer may answer such questions differently at different times. However, reflecting on such questions can help you pursue work that is most consistent with your values.

Once you are pursuing a project, issues beyond the technical can arise in choice of content to include. Some of these issues regard matters such as privacy and taste. Another regards not unduly raising or dashing hopes, given that readers with health conditions are often vulnerable. And another regards engendering due concern about public health problems while avoiding scaremongering. Thoughtfully approaching issues such as these can aid in obtaining suitable balance.

Choice of Employers and Publication Sites

Health writing for the public contains many niches. Your answers to questions about which health writing does good, or does the most good, can help you identify the niches that are most consistent with your values. Given your values and your mix of skills, could you contribute more by writing for the media or by working in public information or public relations? In the media, would it, for example, be better to do television reporting that reaches a broad audience but rarely permits coverage in depth or to write for a newspaper or magazine that allows more thorough coverage but reaches a narrower segment? In the latter case, which segments of the public do you consider most worth reaching? And if you favor public information work, which institutions, and which activities thereof, are most in keeping with your priorities? Would you accomplish most by providing information to the media, preparing materials for the public yourself, or a doing a combination of both? Although of course the job market can limit a health writer's options, considering such questions can aid in deciding which opportunities to pursue.

If you do freelance work, similar questions can arise. For example, for which publications or institutions would it be most worthwhile to write? Are there any you should avoid? For instance, should you refuse to write for magazines that publish cigarette advertising? Or could the good done by the writing outweigh contributing to a publication supported in part by promoting a habit that endangers health?

Of course, while considering such questions health writers may need to be realistic about constraints. Opportunities are sometimes limited, yet bills must still be paid. Sometimes taking work that one values less highly can allow survival as a health writer and continued professional development until better options arise. And income from assignments of lower personal priority can provide financial freedom to write for causes one especially favors. The answers may not be perfect, but raising and considering the questions can aid in choosing the best options.

Conflict of Interest

That health writers should avoid conflicts of interest may seem almost too obvious to state. Clearly health writers for the media should not accept payment or gifts from parties seeking coverage. Writers employed by publications or public information offices should not freelance for competing entities. And when journals contain findings on medical products, health writers should not take advantage of their early copies in buying or selling stocks.

Sometimes, however, possible conflicts of interest are more subtle and less readily avoidable. If you do a student internship in an institution's public relations office, how objectively can you later cover that institution as a health reporter? Or if you do an internship at a media site, will you later favor that site if you work in public information? If you attend a science writers' seminar, will you tend to give the sponsoring association extra coverage? What if you do a mid-career fellowship at a university? Might that bias your coverage in favor of the fellowship site? And what if sources you interview become your friends, as can readily occur over the years as one covers a field such as health?

If you are a health professional as well as a health writer, additional potential can exist for conflict of interest. Can you write objectively about the health professions, or are there topics you should avoid? Might writing for the media give you or your institution unwarranted economic advantage? Where does journalism end and public relations begin? Is there potential to exploit your patients as sources or to neglect them because of your writing? On the other hand, might being a health writer spur you to keep up with the literature more fully and thus help you serve patients bet-

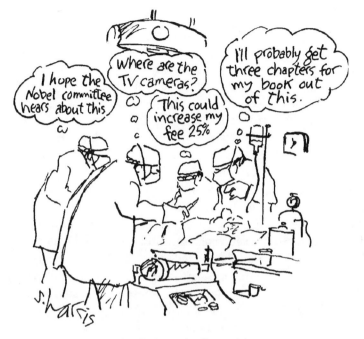

© Sidney Harris, reproduced by permission.

ter? Likewise, as suggested by physician author Perri Klass (1992), might trying to understand patients' experiences in order to write about them make you a more sensitive clinician?

Finally, health can be a highly personal and emotional topic, and health writers can hardly avoid bringing biases from their own backgrounds. For example, diseases that they themselves have experienced, or that have affected those around them, can loom disproportionately large. And many writers have topics in health that they would rather not confront.

In short, any health writer who is a human being probably cannot totally avoid conflicts of interest. However, awareness of possible sources of bias can aid in doing fair and balanced and intellectually honest work. When such awareness may not suffice, one option is to have another writer take on the project in question. Another possibility is simply, in keeping with the principle of truthfulness, to be candid with your audience about possible limitations to your objectivity.

III. Exploring Areas and Issues

Privacy and Confidentiality

For health writers, issues of privacy and confidentiality can arise in at least two contexts. One is writing about the health of public figures such as government officials, athletes, and entertainers. Another is writing about people who themselves may not be of public interest but who have health conditions that are.

On choosing to become a public figure, one relinquishes some privacy. It can well be argued, for example, that the public has a right to know about the president's health. And though doing so should be a matter of choice, public figures can sometimes contribute to public health by disclosing their illnesses, thus engendering publicity that leads to prevention, diagnosis, and treatment in others.

Professional ethics preclude a doctor from releasing information about a patient without the patient's consent. Thus, it is inappropriate to request such information from a public figure's doctor. However, it is appropriate to approach public information staff for information on an ill or injured public figure's health. If such information has been released, it may then be presented by a doctor or other spokesperson.

When writing about private individuals, the issue is often that of distinguishing what one should tell from what one could tell. As noted in the chapter on interviewing, people inexperienced in dealing with the media frequently reveal personal items under the assumption that the items would not appear in print or on the air. Also, health writers who visit people repeatedly to write about the course of an illness may observe many intimate details. Technically, all is fair game in a story unless the source says otherwise in advance. A caring approach, however, requires respect for the person portrayed and thus sensitivity in deciding what to include. When in doubt, one approach is to discuss the decision with the person being portrayed.

Depiction of Disfigurement and Dysfunction

Areas calling for sensitivity include the portrayal of disfigurement and dysfunction. For example, photographs of people with malformations may merely play to voyeurism. The same might be said for photos of people disfigured by injury. However, some have noted, inclusion of such photos can facilitate society's acceptance of people thus affected (Cohen and Morgan 1988, Fry 1988, Klein 1988).

Similarly, mentioning that a person has a symptom such as incontinence may diminish the person's dignity. Yet exclusion of such information may preclude a full and accurate picture of the disease being discussed. One compromise is to avoid saying that the person has the symptom but elsewhere in the piece to list the symptom as among those that can occur.

A number of thoughtful articles have discussed cases entailing such issues and others noted earlier in this chapter. Two (Fry 1988, Klein 1988) focus on coverage of a girl recovering from severe burns. Another (Steele 1992) discusses the writing of a series on a pair of men with AIDS. And another (Garrett 1989) deals with issues arising when journalists chronicle patients' experiences over time. For models of how journalists have approached such issues, such readings are highly recommended.

Use of Media to Garner Resources

A child needs money for an organ transplant. An association devoted to fighting a disease is launching a fundraising event. And the media are being asked to help call forth resources from the community.

Here, it might surely seem, is a chance for the health writer to do good. However, questions of fairness arise. Not everyone needing resources for a costly procedure can receive the media's help in garnering funds; coverage appears to go disproportionately to cute children, candidates with especially dramatic stories, and people whose families are media-savvy. Likewise, not every medical charity event can be covered; sometimes coverage depends not on the impact of the problem being addressed but on the vigor of the event's organizers. Also, questions exist of whether the resources being sought for an individual or cause could do more good if used in other ways.

Here, explicit attention to fairness helps ensure that attention is distributed soundly. Such attention requires looking at the big picture, as encouraged elsewhere in this book, rather than merely reacting to each instance as it occurs. A broad view can yield consistent guidelines on what type of coverage, if any, to give what type of call for resources. And it can promote coverage that, as recommended by various authors (for example, Boisaubin 1988, Smith 1993, Baldwin 1994), considers the larger issues relating to matters such as organ transplants, rather than focusing only on individual people and causes.

III. Exploring Areas and Issues

Participation in Writing Contests

Many awards exist for health writing in general or for writing about specific health topics. In addition, health writers can compete for, and often win, more general prizes for writing or reporting. Examples of awards that may especially interest health writers are listed in Table 12-1. Although this table lists only national awards, regional awards for health writing are available as well.

As a member of the health-writing community, you are likely to receive information on competitions for various awards. Health-related organizations that you have contacted in your work may send you announcements of writing contests they sponsor. Publications and mailings of groups such as the American Medical Writers Association and the National Association of Science Writers contain information on writing competitions. Sponsors of contests sometimes draw on the mailing lists of such associations. If you are seeking information on contests, resources include the journalism awards issue that the magazine *Editor & Publisher* publishes at the end of each year.

But why, you may be wondering, are awards being mentioned in a chapter on ethics? Can recognition of excellence in health writing be anything but good? After all, achievement deserves recognition. The availability of awards may spur health writers to do their best. And receiving an award can encourage a writer to continue striving for high standards. Receipt of awards also can aid in obtaining the opportunities and support needed to accomplish most as a health writer.

The issue is the potential for availability of awards to influence a writer's judgment. Choosing to pursue a story because an award exists for writing about the topic, or gearing a story's content or style to what one thinks judges will like, can conflict with doing what you deem best. Choose to write about what you consider worthwhile, and present the topic as you see fit. If your work happens to qualify for an award competition, do apply if you like. If you win, excellent, so long as the recognition does not bias your future coverage. But better to do writing that meets your values and standards and never win a contest than to compromise your judgment in the successful pursuit of awards. For integrity in choice of topics and content, the first ethical issue discussed in this chapter and one encompassing various others, is essential to being a health writer who not only does well but does good.

Table 12-1: Examples of Awards Available for Health Writing

Award	Contact for Information
AWARDS FOR HEALTH OR SCIENCE WRITING IN GENERAL	
AAAS Science Journalism Awards (note: entries may be on biomedical research but not solely on health or clinical medicine)	American Association for the Advancement of Science Office of Communications 1200 New York Avenue, NW Washington DC 20005 phone: (202) 326-6431
AIBS Media Award (for reporting on research in biology; entries may be on basic biomedical research but not on testing of medical treatments)	AIBS Media Award American Institute of Biological Sciences 1444 I Street, NW Suite 200 Washington, DC 20005 phone: (202) 628-1500, Ext. 206
AMWA Medical Book Awards (categories: books for physicians, books for allied health professionals, books for the lay public)	American Medical Writers Association Book Awards Committee 9650 Rockville Pike Bethesda, Maryland 20814 phone: (301) 493-0003
Evert Clark Award (for science journalists age 30 or below; print media only)	Evert Clark Fund National Press Foundation 529 14th Street, NW Washington, DC 20045 phone: (202) 662-7350
International Health and Medical Film Competition (Freddie Awards)	International Health and Medical Film Competition 24050 Madison Street, Suite 104 Torrance, California 90505 phone: (310) 791-6616
Jules Bergman Award (for a program by a National Association of Physician Broadcasters member)	National Association of Physician Broadcasters 515 North State Street, 12th Floor Chicago, Illinois 60610 phone: (312) 464-5852
National Health Information Awards (largely for materials produced by organizations)	Health Information Resource Center 621 East Park Avenue Libertyville, Illinois 60048 phone: (800) 828-8225

Table 12-1:   Awards (*continued*)

Science-in-Society
Journalism Awards

National Association of Science Writers
P.O. Box 294
Greenlawn, New York 11740
phone: (516) 757-5664

American College of
Allergy, Asthma and
Immunology National
Media Awards

Public Relations Director
American College of Allergy, Asthma
    and Immunology
85 West Algonquin Road, Suite 550
Arlington Heights, Illinois 60005
phone: (847) 427-1200

American Podiatric
Medical Association
Journalism Awards

American Podiatric Medical Association
9312 Old Georgetown Road
Bethesda, Maryland 20814
phone: (301) 581-9227

American Society of
Colon and Rectal
Surgeons National
Media Awards

American Society of Colon and
    Rectal Surgeons
85 West Algonquin Road, Suite 550
Arlington Heights, Illinois 60005
phone: (847) 290-9184

ASHA National Media
Awards

Communication Department
American Speech-Language-Hearing
    Association
10801 Rockville Pike
Rockville, Maryland 20852
phone: (301) 897-5700

ASM Public Communications
Award (for stories on
microbiology)

American Society for Microbiology
1325 Massachusetts Avenue, NW
Washington, DC 20005
phone: (202) 942-9297

"Breaking the Mold" Award
for Innovation and
Excellence in Media
Coverage of Plastic
Surgery

Media Relations Manager
American Society of Plastic
    and Reconstructive Surgeons
444 East Algonquin Road
Arlington Heights, Illinois 60005
phone: (847) 228-9900, Ext. 347

Epilepsy Foundation
of America Distinguished
Journalism Award

Epilepsy Foundation of America
4351 Garden City Drive
Landover, Maryland 20785
phone: (301) 459-3700

Table 12-1: *(continued)*

Leukemia Society of America Annual Journalism Awards	Marketing and Communications Department Leukemia Society of America 600 3rd Avenue, 4th Floor New York, New York 10016 phone: (212) 573-8484
Media Excellence Awards (for writing about mental retardation)	The Arc 500 East Border Street, Suite 300 Arlington, Texas 76010 phone: (817) 261-6003
MS Public Education Awards (for reporting on multiple sclerosis)	Public Affairs Department National Multiple Sclerosis Society 733 3rd Avenue, 6th Floor New York, New York 10017 phone: (212) 986-3240
National Easter Seal EDI [Equality, Dignity, and Independence] Award (for media efforts regarding people with disabilities)	National Easter Seal Society 230 West Monroe Street, Suite 1800 Chicago, Illinois 60606 phone: (312) 726-6200
National Mental Health Association Mental Health Media Awards	National Mental Health Association 1021 Prince Street Alexandria, Virginia 22314 phone: (703) 838-7528
PAHO Excellence in International Public Health Reporting Awards	Pan American Health Organization 525 23rd Street, NW Washington, DC 20037 phone: (202) 974-3457
Pat Weaver/MDA Award (for broadcast productions on neuromuscular diseases)	Muscular Dystrophy Association Inc. 3300 East Sunrise Drive Tucson, Arizona 85718 (520) 529-2000
Planned Parenthood Federation of America Maggie Awards Program	Planned Parenthood Federation of America 810 Seventh Avenue New York, New York 10019 phone: (212) 261-4650

Table 12-1: **Awards (*continued*)**

Primary Care Journalism Awards	UCSF Center for the Health Professions 1388 Sutter Street, Suite 805 San Francisco, California 94109 phone: (415) 476-8181
Ray Bruner Science Writing Award (for writing related to public health; restricted to reporters with limited experience)	Public Relations Director American Public Health Association 1015 15th Street, NW, Suite 300 Washington, DC 20005 phone: (202) 789-5677
Robert L. Robinson Award (broadcast) and Robert T. Morse Award (print) for coverage of mental illness	Division of Public Affairs American Psychiatric Association 1400 K Street, NW Washington, DC 20005 phone: (202) 682-6142
Rosa Cisneros Memorial Information Prize (for family planning/population information in the Western Hemisphere)	Communications Office International Planned Parenthood Federation Western Hemisphere Region 120 Wall Street, 9th Floor New York, New York 10005 phone: (212) 248-6400
Rose Kushner Award (for writing about breast cancer)	American Medical Writers Association 9650 Rockville Pike Bethesda, Maryland 20814 phone: (301) 493-0003
Russell L. Cecil Arthritis Medical Journalism Awards	Public Relations Arthritis Foundation 1330 West Peachtree Street Atlanta, Georgia 30309 phone: (404) 872-7100
Stuttering Foundation of America Reporting Excellence on Stuttering Award	Stuttering Foundation of America P.O. Box 11749 Memphis, Tennessee 38111 phone: (800) 992-9392

SOURCES: *Editor & Publisher*, 30 December 1995 and 28 December 1996; announcements from contest sponsors.
NOTE: Awards sometimes are discontinued. Contact parties listed for information on current availability.

PART IV

Pursuing a Career

Chapter 13

(ARÉÉR OPTIONS

Mention health writing, and many people think only of newspaper medical reporting. However, as shown by the classified advertisements excerpted in Figure 13-1, health writing includes many options: jobs in various media old and new, positions in public information for various institutions, and various types of freelance work. This chapter describes major options and discusses pursuing them. Realize, though, that given the increasingly varied ways that health information is presented, you may find yourself doing work of types not imagined.

Media Old and New

Health writing for the media is a growing niche in at least two ways. First, the scope of what health writers cover has expanded. Until recently health writing generally was mainly medical writing, focusing largely on medical advances and tending to look uncritically at the world of medicine. Today, however, health writing looks increasingly at issues relating to health and takes the more skeptical stance traditional in journalism. Second, with the growth of health newsletters and the advent of new computerized media, additional opportunities have emerged.

Larger newspapers commonly have health writers, as do wire services (for example, the Associated Press). At smaller newspapers, the same person may cover both science and health, or health may be part of a general reporter's beat. Many health writers began as general reporters and moved—or were cast—into the health writer role. However, especially at the largest newspapers, some health writers have science backgrounds or were trained as health professionals. As well as preparing their own stories, health writers at newspapers and news magazines sometimes serve as consultants to other staff members whose stories have a medical aspect.

Although many magazines depend largely on freelancers for medical stories, some, such as the news weeklies, have health or medical writers on their staffs. Opportunities for employment also exist at popular magazines that focus on health or science, at magazines for health professionals, and

Figure 13-1: **Excerpts from Some Recent Announcements of Jobs for Health Writers**

Health-Medical Reporter. Award-winning 60,000-circulation newspaper in Big Ten University community is seeking an aggressive reporter with experience covering health care/medical/science issues. Must be able to translate cutting-edge medical research into stories that the non-Ph.D. reader can understand. . . . (*Editor & Publisher*)

Medical Writer. The *State Journal-Register* . . . seeks an experienced medical writer. Successful applicant will have proven record in covering state and national health trends, local news, and a thorough understanding of technical, consumer and fitness issues. Assignment also includes in-depth reporting for a weekly health section. . . . (*American Medical Writers Association Job Market Sheet*)

Reporter. The *Post-Dispatch* is looking for a reporter to cover health care. . . . We're looking for someone who will write compelling stories about real people; explain complex issues clearly and engagingly; write features and spot news; enjoy breaking news; develop sources; generate story ideas; use government and hospital and court records to help readers assess the quality of HMOs, hospitals, doctors and other health-care providers; know how to analyze databases and explore the Internet and online services. . . . (*American Medical Writers Association Job Market Sheet*)

Editor—Northwest Health. Group Health Cooperative, the Northwest's pre-eminent managed-healthcare system, seeks an editor for *Northwest Health*, its 260,000-circulation member magazine, published six times a year. . . . (*Editor & Publisher*)

Medical Writer/Editor. . . . For our new . . . newsletter, *HealthNews*, we are seeking a Medical Writer/Editor with extensive experience in medical news writing for a lay audience who has published on a wide variety of health topics. . . . (*Science-Writers*)

Medical Research Writer/Editor—U.S. Dept. of Veterans Affairs. . . . The writer/editor's primary responsibility will be to prepare stories and news releases concerning research occurring at VA medical centers. The candidate must be able to interview scientists and clinical investigators about their research and compose articles that are understandable for the medically naive reader. . . . (*Hiring Line*)

Specialist, Public Relations. Children's National Medical Center has an opening for a specialist, public relations. The position involves writing and editing health and science related press releases, organizing and presenting special events at the hospital, researching and pitching pro-active story ideas to local and national media outlets and responding to media inquiries. . . . (*ASHCMPR/SHPM Career Opportunities Bulletin*)

Medical/Science Writer. . . . Roswell Park Cancer Institute, the nation's first and one of its largest cancer research and treatment centers, is seeking a medical/science writer who enjoys media placement challenges. Applicants should have at

Figure 13-1: *(continued)*

least 3 years experience, preferably as a medical/science journalist or in a news bureau operation. . . . (*Hiring Line*)

Writer/Editor. . . . Write/edit publications for major patient-care and biomedical research institution (including newsletter, annual report, patient brochures, and other editorial projects as they arise). Coordinate editing/production of major research report and symposium abstract books. Contribute to and ultimately oversee editorial production of institution's Internet website. . . . Solid science background and journalism and/or PR experience required. . . . (*American Medical Writers Association Job Market Sheet*)

Medical/Science Writer. Penn State University's College of Medicine and hospitals at the Milton S. Hershey Medical Center is recruiting energetic and experienced writer and publicist. This is primarily a writing position—in-depth science and medical articles written for national media outlets and the Medical Center's magazine. . . . (*American Medical Writers Association Job Market Sheet*)

Manager, News Media Relations. The American Heart Association, National Center, seeks a manager of News Media Relations to direct national news media operations. Activities include contact with news media, writing, editing, and promoting the flow of news and other AHA related information to the media. . . . (*Science-Writers*)

Science Writer. The Office of Public Affairs of a scientific society representing 25,000 members seeks a versatile science writer. . . . Responsibilities include reporting and writing news releases, planning press events and conferences, and preparing a news column on issues affecting science and newsletter articles explaining the importance of basic neuroscience research. . . . (*Science*)

Medical Writer. Healthwise, Inc., located in Boise, Idaho, has full-time positions available for medical writers. . . . Writers at HealthWise translate complex medical information into consumer-friendly language to help medical consumers make well-informed decisions about their health. . . . (*American Medical Writers Association Job Market Sheet*)

Editor/Medical Writer. The nation's largest publisher for conventions is seeking an experienced medical communications specialist to join the editorial team in writing, editing and producing on-site daily publications at the nation's leading medical association meetings. . . . (*American Medical Writers Association Job Market Sheet*)

Freelance Writer, Medical News. The *British Medical Journal* . . . is seeking to recruit news correspondents in the U.S., Canada and Mexico to help monitor, collect, and prepare news items for each week's *BMJ*. . . . (*American Medical Writers Association Job Market Sheet*) in the news sections of some medical and scientific journals. Some health writers work for institutional magazines, such as those published by medical schools or health maintenance organizations.

Broadcast media draw on people with various backgrounds for their health reporting. In recent years, physicians working full-time or, more commonly, part-time for the media have delivered a substantial amount of the medical news on television. However, staff from broadcast-journalism and other backgrounds continue to do much health coverage on the air and work behind the scenes. Although radio appears to have few health reporters, some exist, for example, at National Public Radio.

Health newsletters, which vary in their proportions of staff and freelance work, are an additional niche for health writers. Over the past decade or so, these newsletters have multiplied, reaching more than 30. They now include not only such general publications as the *Harvard Health Letter*, the *University of California at Berkeley Wellness Letter*, and the *Mayo Clinic Health Letter* but also specialized newsletters in areas such as nutrition, mental health, and women's health (Hamlin 1995).

New electronic media also offer opportunities for health writers—and promise to offer more. Thus, health writers with needed technical skills

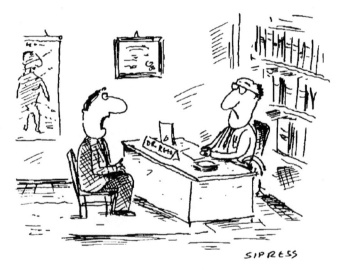

**"I want to have that operation I heard about
on *All Things Considered*."**

may well be in high demand by companies such as those that produce multimedia products. Among other media employing health writers are museums and book publishers. The possibilities are varied indeed.

Public Information and Public Relations

A considerable proportion of health writers work in public information or public relations. Sites of employment include universities, government agencies, pharmaceutical and other companies, voluntary health organizations such as the American Diabetes Association and the American Lung Association, professional societies, and health-care facilities. Some health writers work for public relations agencies or for consulting firms that prepare materials on health for various institutions or companies.

Commonly, PI and PR offices of health-related institutions both produce writing and provide information for other writers. If you are the sole person in such an office, or one of only a few, you may have a considerable mix of duties. In some larger offices, however, your duties may be highly specialized. Before seeking a position, you may wish to consider what sort of range you prefer.

In a public information or public relations office, you may do various kinds of health writing. You may prepare written news releases for dissemination in print or electronically; if you have a broadcasting background, you may prepare video news releases. You may produce brochures, fact sheets, videotapes, and other materials for the public. You may write media backgrounders, magazine or newsletter articles, and speeches. You may produce newsletters or magazines. You may be responsible as well for publications such as annual reports. Your work may include producing material for use on the World Wide Web. Both journalists and the public may draw on the writing you do.

Alternatively or in addition, you may provide material specifically for others' writing in any of various ways. Your role may include answering questions from reporters and recommending expert sources to interview. You may provide graphics or videotape for use by the media. If major news arises, you may be responsible for arranging a press conference. Your work may include setting up the news room or otherwise assisting reporters at conferences your institution holds. You may arrange activities such as science writers' seminars to brief members of the media.

In some offices, you may also be responsible for answering questions directly from the public. Your role may include arranging and publicizing public-education events. You may also train researchers or others at your institution in working effectively with the media. And especially if you are in a leadership position, you may develop strategies for disseminating information.

How can you prepare for such a niche? Emily N. Avila, who works in public information at the University of California at Davis medical school, says: "Be a reporter first." She finds that having been a television reporter helps her understand and meet reporters' needs. "I can anticipate their questions, which makes it easier for me to prepare our experts for interviews," she says, "and their other needs, such as B roll for TV or finding a patient to add a personal touch."

Others in the field—often those working mainly in writing rather than media relations—arrive at their positions through other routes. Backgrounds include journalism, science, and sometimes the health professions. In public information and public relations, as in health writing in general, many paths to success exist.

Freelance Writing

For health writers, freelance opportunities abound. Magazines and newsletters are always seeking health writers who produce first-rate work and deliver it promptly. And many public relations and public information offices draw on freelancers to prepare written or audiovisual materials.

Some health writers do only freelance work, either by choice or while seeking other employment. Others freelance to supplement the income or experience provided by their jobs. Employers vary in their policies and attitudes toward freelancing. In any event, ethics require avoiding conflicts of interest.

Freelancing full time can have advantages and disadvantages. You can keep largely the hours of your choice and can work out of your home. If demand for your work is high, you can choose among assignments. You do not have a boss (or you have various bosses, some of whom you can choose not to work for again if you have enough else to do). And, one freelancer says with relief, "I never have to wear pantyhose."

On the other hand, full-time freelancing takes discipline. It also can be lonely. It does not offer benefits, such as insurance, that employers commonly supply. You generally must provide your own office equipment, and you may spend considerable time marketing your work and otherwise running your business, rather than writing about health.

Launching a freelance career tends to be easier once you have been employed. You have more experience, more credentials, and more contacts; quite likely, you also have more money to draw on in case income is slow in arriving. If freelance opportunities in health writing per se are limited at first, consider accepting related work, such as biomedically related technical writing or editing.

Magazines are a major outlet for freelance health writing. Do not only consider magazines focusing on health or science; many other magazines—such as women's magazines, trade (occupational) magazines, and local or regional magazines—run articles on health. Listings of many of the magazines publishing freelance work appear in the annual guide *Writer's Market* (Holm 1996). This guide also includes information on markets other than magazines (for example, book publishers) and advice on freelance writing.

Though listings in *Writer's Market* can be fine starting points, they do not suffice. To propose and prepare an appropriate story, you must know a magazine well. Often, the magazines you will write for best are those you enjoy reading. Whatever the magazine, before seeking an assignment consider questions such as the following: For whom is the magazine intended? (Here, advertisements as well as articles can provide useful clues.) What is the writing style? How long are the articles? What sections or departments does the magazine have, and where might your writing fit? On what areas do the health pieces tend to focus? For example, does the magazine run mainly articles on healthy living? diseases and their management? medical research? health policy?

To assist authors, many magazines prepare writer's guidelines. These guidelines commonly indicate what sorts of work the magazine is seeking and how to prepare and submit it. Write to the magazine to request such guidelines; enclose a stamped, self-addressed envelope. Also look for guidelines posted on the World Wide Web.

With rare exceptions, magazines request (or require) that authors contact them beforehand about possible assignments rather than proceeding to submit finished articles. Traditionally, such contact is made via a "query letter"—that is, a letter describing the story you propose and noting your credentials to write it; typically such a letter runs about one page and is accompanied by examples of articles you have published. An alternative, especially if your background would make you especially attractive to the magazine, is to inform the editor of your availability; if interested, the editor may then ask you for story ideas or assign a piece on a topic of his or her choosing. Once you have established a strong working relationship with an editor, interchange of ideas often becomes more informal.

Other advice on magazine writing: Consider starting small. For example, begin by proposing a brief piece for the health news section of a magazine; writing such pieces well can help you win assignments for long feature stories. Also, retain your source materials for use in your own fact checking and that by members of the magazine staff. If you have not taken a magazine writing class, consider doing so or looking at some of the many books available on magazine writing. Also consider scanning magazines such as *Writer's Digest* and *The Writer*, which often include practical advice on magazine writing. For information on payment and other business aspects of freelance writing for magazines and other media, consult such resources as *Writer's Market*, the *National Writers Union Guide to Freelance Rates and Standard Practice* (Kopelman 1995), and fellow freelancers.

Finally, keep good financial records on your freelance writing. Be sure to save the information you need to compute your income tax; also retain the documentation required for the tax breaks to which you are entitled. Speaking of breaks: Beware of some freelancers' tendencies to work day and night and never turn down a project. Know your limits, and take the breaks you need to maintain your own health.

Finding Health-Writing Opportunities

In the media, public information, and the freelance sector, many health-writing opportunities exist. But how can you find them? Approaches include reading job announcements, networking, and simply taking the initiative to inquire.

Some classified advertisements for health-writing opportunities appear in general newspapers. In addition, consult more specialized publications and listings. For example, if you seek a newspaper health-writing job, look at classified advertisements in the trade magazine *Editor & Publisher*. If you wish to work in an academic setting or for an association, look at such advertisements in the *Chronicle of Higher Education*, and if possible follow the weekly listings in Hiring Line, an online job-listing service available to institutions that are members of ProfNet (http://www.profnet.com). Should you lack access to Hiring Line yourself, see whether a colleague working in a university (or other) public information office subscribing to this service will share the listings.

13. Career Options

Consult the American Medical Writers Association (AMWA) job market sheet, which is published nine times per year and includes both full-time and freelance opportunities. Read the classified advertisements in the National Association of Science Writers (NASW) newsletter, *ScienceWriters*.

In addition, network, network, network. Join organizations such as AMWA and NASW. Get to know fellow members, who may be aware of job openings—and may keep you in mind when they have staff to hire or freelance projects to assign. Consult professors who know you and may be able to help, and look at postings in schools or departments of journalism. Let it be widely known that you are seeking work; job leads and freelance opportunities often materialize from unexpected sources. Take freelance or volunteer projects that may increase your visibility. If you are beginning your career or changing fields, consider doing an internship, which may lead to a job or provide the experience and contacts to get one. Especially if you are more experienced, consider consulting an employment agency, particularly one with special strength in the communications or health field.

Even if openings are not announced, contact sites for which you might like to work. More than one health writer has landed a job or freelance work in this way. Even if a site has no work to offer, the contact you make may direct you to opportunities elsewhere.

Many varied opportunities exist in health writing, and there are many ways to find them. But how can you prepare yourself for such opportunities and stay up-to-date? Such questions are among those addressed in the next two chapters, which deal with professional organizations and educational opportunities.

Chapter 14

PROFESSIONAL ORGANIZATIONS

Health writing can be a lonely profession. Generally only one health writer works at a media site or institution. Even major health publications and public information offices of major medical institutions often have small professional staffs. The reality is that freelance health writing is largely a solitary pursuit.

Professional organizations, such as the American Medical Writers Association and the National Association of Science Writers, can help overcome health writers' isolation. Not only do such organizations offer fellowship and opportunity to exchange ideas, but through their meetings and publications, they also offer information important in staying up to date and advancing in one's career.

This chapter introduces professional organizations for health writers and members of related fields. Students reading the chapter should note that some of these organizations offer student memberships at a reduced rate. If such memberships are not announced, feel free to ask about them.

Main Organizations

American Medical Writers Association
Founded: 1940
Membership: about 4,000
Address: 9650 Rockville Pike
    Bethesda, Maryland 20814-3998
Phone: (301) 493-0003
Fax: (301) 493-6384
E-Mail: amwa@amwa.org
World Wide Web: http://www.amwa.org/amwa

The American Medical Writers Association (AMWA) serves members specializing in health writing and other areas of biomedical communication. Many members work for educational or other institutions, for the pharmaceutical industry, or as freelance writers or editors; relatively few are reporters for daily media. The organization's scope is reflected by the names of its sections: Editing/Writing, Freelance, Public Relations/Advertising/Marketing, Pharmaceutical, Audiovisual, and Educators.

AMWA holds an annual conference, generally in late October or early November; it also presents regional workshops and conferences. In addition, it publishes the *AMWA Journal*, the *AMWA Freelance Directory*, the *AMWA Membership Directory*, and the *AMWA Job Market Sheet*. AMWA also has published two books presenting highlights of selected AMWA workshops (Minick 1994, Witte and Taylor 1997). As well as 17 regional chapters in the United States, AMWA has a Canadian chapter and a European chapter.

Education is a major emphasis of AMWA. The annual conference typically includes more than 70 workshops. By completing designated numbers and distributions of workshops, AMWA members can earn certificates. Different workshops serve different professional interests in AMWA; most of the workshops are intended to help develop professional skills, but some are meant to increase participants' biomedical knowledge. Among titles of repeatedly offered workshops likely to interest many health writers are Bibliographic Resources for Medical Communicators, Anatomy and Physiology for Poets, Effective Interviewing, Improving Comprehension: Theories and Research Findings, Newsletter Production, Writing a Health-Related Book Proposal and Doing Your Own PR, and Business Aspects of a Freelance Career.

National Association of Science Writers
Founded: 1934
Membership: about 1,800
Address: P.O. Box 294
        Greenlawn, New York 11740
Phone: (516) 757-5664
Fax: (516) 757-0069
E-Mail: diane@nasw.org
World Wide Web: http://www.nasw.org

Founded by a dozen pioneering science reporters, the National Association of Science Writers (NASW) now numbers more than 1,800 members. About half are employed by the media or freelance full time; most of the rest work in public relations or public information. Of members listed in a recent directory, about half designated health, medicine, or both as among their areas of specialty.

14. Professional Organizations

Over the years, the NASW newsletter, *ScienceWriters*, has been an excellent resource. Articles in this quarterly newsletter often deal with health writing. The newsletter serves well for keeping up with issues, trends, and happenings in health writing and science writing. NASW also has published a 34-page primer titled *Communicating Science News: A Guide for Public Information Officers, Scientists and Physicians* (1996).

In addition, NASW has prepared a science-writing book, *A Field Guide for Science Writers* (Blum and Knudson 1997), for use by students and young reporters. It includes chapters on aspects of health writing. The NASW also publishes a membership directory.

NASW meets each winter in conjunction with the American Association for Advancement of Science national meeting, which many science writers cover. Until recent years, NASW held little more than a business meeting and social gathering. Now, however, NASW offers a substantial educational program. Topics of workshops have included Internet resources and their use, interaction between reporters and government agencies, and means other than news releases to promote university research.

Although NASW does not have regional chapters per se, it does have local affiliates. Areas with such science writers groups have included New England, Northern California, and the District of Columbia. The contact people for these groups change periodically; current information can be obtained from NASW.

National Association of Physician Broadcasters
Founded: 1982
Membership: about 250
Address: 515 North State Street
Chicago, Illinois 60610
Phone: (312) 464-5852
Fax: (312) 464-5843

The National Association of Physician Broadcasters (NAPB) is an organization mainly of physicians working in the electronic and print media. The NAPB has members in more than 40 states and several foreign countries. It has a close working relationship with the American Medical Association.

With the AMA, the NAPB sponsors two conferences per year: the AMA Health Reporting Conference, usually held in the spring, and the AMA

IV.   Pursuing a Career

Science Reporters Conference, in the fall. NAPB publishes a quarterly newsletter and a membership directory. Members receive announcements of media briefings and are alerted to videotaped and printed materials available for use in their work.

Any physician or dentist interested in participating in medical media may apply for medical membership in the NAPB. Associate memberships are available to members of other health professions and to journalists who are not health professionals.

Organizations in Related Areas

Associations in areas related to medical or science writing also can be resources for health writers. Information on such organizations is provided below.

Society of Environmental Journalists
Founded: 1990
Membership: about 1,100
Address: P.O. Box 27280
   Philadelphia, Pennsylvania 19118
Phone: (215) 836-9970
Fax: (215) 836-9972
E-Mail: SEJOffice@aol.com
World Wide Web: http://www.sej.org

Programs and services of the Society of Environmental Journalists (SEJ) include national conferences, regional seminars, and the *SEJournal*, a quarterly newsletter. Often the conference sessions or newsletter articles address health-related topics. Journalists and academicians can join SEJ; public relations professionals cannot be members but can subscribe to the newsletter and attend the conferences.

Council of Biology Editors Inc.
Founded: 1957
Membership: about 1,200
Address: 60 Revere Drive, Suite 500
   Northbrook, Illinois 60062
Phone: (847) 480-6349

14. Professional Organizations

Fax: (847) 480-9282
E-Mail: cbehdqts@aol.com
World Wide Web: http://www.sdsc.edu/CBE

Although the Council of Biology Editors (CBE) focuses mainly on the editing of scholarly writing in science and medicine, its activities and publications also can aid those who do popular health writing. CBE holds an annual meeting and offers retreats and short courses. It also publishes a newsletter, *CBE Views*, as well as books on topics relating to biology editing. Subjects of conference sessions and newsletter articles have included science and the media. CBE membership may especially interest health writers who do scholarly as well as popular writing or editing.

Broader Organizations

Various more general communications organizations can also be good resources for health writers. Among those to consider are the International Association of Business Communicators (IABC), Investigative Reporters and Editors (IRE), the Public Relations Society of America (PRSA), the Society of Professional Journalists (SPJ), and the Society for Technical Communication (STC).

International Association of Business Communicators
Founded: 1970
Membership: about 12,000
Address: One Hallidie Plaza, Suite 600
   San Francisco, California 94102
Phone: (415) 433-3400
Fax: (415) 362-8762
E-Mail: service_centre@iabc.com
World Wide Web: http://www.iabc.com/homepage.htm

Investigative Reporters and Editors
Founded: 1975
Membership: about 3,500
Address: 138 Neff Annex
   University of Missouri School of Journalism
   Columbia, Missouri 65211

IV.   Pursuing a Career

Phone: (573) 882-2042
Fax: (573) 882-5431
E-Mail: jourire@muccmail.missouri.edu
World Wide Web: http://www.ire.org
Comment: For further information, see the section "Investigative and Depth Reporting" in Chapter 8.

Public Relations Society of America
Founded: 1947
Membership: about 17,500
Address: 33 Irving Place
   New York, New York 10003-2376
Phone: (212) 995-2230
Fax: (212) 995-0757
E-Mail: hdq@prsa.org
World Wide Web: http://www.prsa.org
Comment: PRSA includes a professional interest section, the Health Academy, for members working in health care public relations.

Society of Professional Journalists
Founded: 1909
Membership: about 13,500
Address: 16 South Jackson Street
   Greencastle, Indiana 46135
Phone: (765) 653-3333
Fax: (765) 653-4631
E-Mail: spj@link2000.net
World Wide Web: http://www.spj.org

Society for Technical Communication
Founded: 1953
Membership: about 20,000
Address: 901 North Stuart Street, Suite 904
   Arlington, Virginia 22203-1854
Phone: (703) 522-4114
Fax: (703) 522-2075
E-Mail: stc@stc-va.org
World Wide Web: http://www.stc-va.org

14. Professional Organizations

Though many health writers work alone, health writing need not be a lonely profession. Consider joining professional organizations in the field. Not only will you feel less isolated, you also will learn of career opportunities. Perhaps most important, the information you gain can make you a better health writer.

Chapter 15

EDUCATIONAL OPPORTUNITIES

Health writers come from a wide range of backgrounds. More important, superb health writers come from a wide range of backgrounds. These backgrounds include journalism, science, and the health professions; some of the best health writers have studied more than one of these fields. The issue is not what background you start with but how you round it out and how you stay up to date.

As well as learning on the job and through professional organizations, you can increase your health-writing knowledge and skill through courses and degree programs, internships, and fellowships. This chapter focuses on such educational opportunities. Although it emphasizes those opportunities specifically in health writing or science writing, it also discusses more general opportunities from which health writers can benefit.

Courses and Programs

College and university courses in health or science, in journalism and related fields, and specifically in health writing or science writing can aid health writers and health-writers-to-be. In addition, degree or certificate programs in science writing and related areas supply intensive preparation.

Science, Health, and Communication Courses

More and more, it appears, employers of health writers favor candidates with both solid science backgrounds and strong communication skills. Thus, if you are still pursuing a degree, try to plan accordingly. If you have already graduated, consider returning for one or more courses in such fields.

To be best prepared as a health writer, try to study science subjects ranging from the molecular to the population level. Possibilities along this spectrum include biochemistry, cell biology, anatomy (which deals with body structure), physiology (which deals with body function), and epidemiology (which deals with disease distribution in the population). Among other areas useful to study are microbiology (the study of microorganisms), genetics, and nutrition. In addition, courses on topics such as the health care system, human diseases, and environmental health can be of value. If you have graduated and wish to take several such courses, consider pursuing a master's degree in public health.

Try to obtain a solid grounding in study design and statistics. Among courses that can offer such grounding are those in epidemiology, statistics, and research methods. If possible, take a statistics course that focuses on sound reasoning about information rather than one that emphasizes number crunching. If you do not take such a course, read a book with a similar emphasis. Such books include *A Mathematician Reads the Newspaper* (Paulos 1995) and *Seeing Through Statistics* (Utts 1996); the latter includes many examples from areas health writers cover.

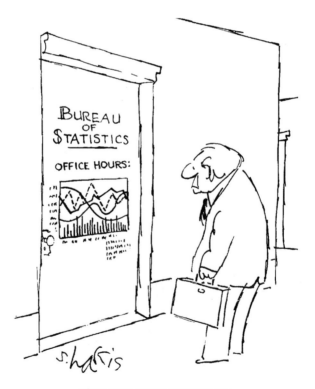

© Sidney Harris, reproduced by permission.

15. Educational Opportunities

Not only credit-bearing courses but also non-credit programs can provide helpful biomedical background. Such programs include the "mini-med schools" (Stephenson 1996) that many medical schools and other biomedical institutions have launched in recent years. Intended to teach the public about medical science, mini-med schools can be a good resource for current and future health writers.

Various classes in journalism or communications can assist you as a health writer. In addition to basic courses in reporting, courses well worth considering include those in information gathering, depth or investigative reporting, magazine writing, and public relations. Even if you do not plan a broadcasting career, consider taking a course in broadcast journalism; the versatility may well increase your marketability, and if you work in media relations, knowing how broadcast media function can increase your effectiveness. Other useful areas of study include graphics and the new electronic media. And, as one young health writer suggests, consider taking a course in medical terminology.

Courses and Programs in Health and Science Writing

Courses and programs specifically in health writing or science writing can help you integrate your learning from science courses and communication courses, as well as develop knowledge and skills specific to health writing and related realms. They also can help you obtain internships and jobs in health-writing. Many of these educational opportunities are described in the *Directory of Science Communication Courses and Programs in the United States* (Dunwoody, Crane, and Brown 1996).

Various colleges and universities offer undergraduate or graduate health-writing courses, at least occasionally. Some of these courses aim mainly to help students develop health-writing skills; others focus largely on analyzing the coverage of health. Science writing courses, which are much more common than courses specifically in health writing, often include material on writing about medicine and health.

Although no major degree programs solely in popular health writing appear to exist, master's degree programs in science writing offer the opportunity to specialize in writing about health. Schools with such programs include Boston University, New York University, The Johns Hopkins University, and Texas A&M University. Another major training ground for science and health journalists is the University of California, Santa Cruz, Science Communication Program; entrance requirements for this three-term certificate program include a science degree and research experience. Also, some highly regarded general graduate programs in journalism—such as those at the University of California-Berkeley, the University of Missouri, and the University of Wisconsin-Madison—offer the opportunity for students to specialize in science writing and, thus, to subspecialize in health writing.

As well as seeking financial aid from their institutions, graduate students wishing to specialize in science writing may apply for support of up to $2,000 from the Council for the Advancement of Science Writing, Inc. Inquiries about applying for these fellowships should be directed to CASW at P.O. Box 404, Greenlawn, New York 11740, telephone (516) 757-5664.

The International Communication Association and the Speech Communication Association recently developed a brochure on programs in health communication (a broad area that deals not only with health journalism but also, for example, with public health campaigns and patient-doctor interactions). Various degree programs and courses may interest prospective or current health writers. The brochure may be obtained from Kim Witte, Michigan State University, telephone (517) 355-9659, e-mail wittek@pilot.msu.edu.

Internships and Related Opportunities

Internships, in which students gain practical experience at a health-writing work site, are a common part of graduate programs in science writing. In addition, freestanding internships are available to students or recent graduates.

"*Please* stress the value of internships," a current graduate student states. "Now I know what the workplace is like and know how to wrap up my degree. I have a job waiting if I want it, as well."

Internships with a health emphasis include the National Cancer Institute graduate internships in health communications. Open to students enrolled in graduate programs, these internships offer opportunities to work in the institute's press section, to write fact sheets and brochures for the public and patients, or to obtain experience in other aspects of cancer communication. Information may be obtained from the Internship Director, Office of Cancer Communications, National Cancer Institute, 31 Center Drive, MSC 2580, Bethesda, Maryland 20892-2580, telephone (301) 496-4394.

Among other sites that have offered science-writing or health-writing internships are *JAMA* (in Chicago), *Science News* and *Science* (in Washing-

15. Educational Opportunities

ton, DC), the Cancer Research Institute (in New York City), and various health-related associations. In addition, health-writing internships are available at hospitals and pharmaceutical companies. Faculty who teach science writing or health writing often know of local and other internships. Also, contacting a publication or public information office where you may wish to do an internship may disclose an opening or lead to the creation of one.

The Business Press Educational Foundation offers an internship program for advanced undergraduates and master's degree students. Through this program, students spend the summer working for publications that target various occupational groups. Among possibilities available are publications for health care professionals. Information on the program can be obtained by calling (212) 661-6360, Ext. 319.

If your background is in science, consider applying for the American Association for the Advancement of Science Mass Media Science and Engineering Fellows Program. This program offers 15 to 20 summer internships per year at newspapers, magazines, and broadcast media. Applicants must be advanced students pursuing degrees in natural or social science, engineering, or the health professions; students in fields such as journalism, science writing, and English are not eligible. Since the program began in 1975, more than 300 fellows, most of them graduate students, have participated. Many subsequently have pursued careers in science writing or have combined science-communication work with other careers. Information on the program is available from the Coordinator, AAAS Mass Media Science and Engineering Fellows Program, 1200 New York Avenue, NW, Washington, DC 20005, telephone (202) 326-6760.

The American Association for Microbiology Student Science Journalism Honors Program especially favors applicants who are graduate students in science writing. Participants in this three-day program, held in the spring in Washington, DC, meet with scientists, public policy officials, and science journalists. Information and applications may be obtained from the Office of Communications, American Society for Microbiology, 1325 Massachusetts Avenue, NW, Washington, DC 20005, telephone (202) 942-9297, fax (202) 942-9367, e-mail communications@asmusa.org.

Fellowships

Various mid-career and other fellowships provide health writers and others with the opportunity to pursue nondegree study or work on special projects. Some of the fellowships are specifically in medical writing or science writing; others are more general. A number that may especially interest health writers are described here.

In 1995 the Reuter Foundation announced a pair of medical-journalism fellowships, one at Columbia University in New York City and one at Oxford University in England. Each fellowship permits an experienced medical writer or broadcaster to spend one academic term studying current medical issues, developments, or trends. Information on the Reuter Fellowship in Medical Journalism may be obtained from the Office of the Dean, Columbia University Graduate School of Journalism, New York, New York 10027, telephone (212) 854-3862.

The Kaiser Media Fellowships Program in Health, established in 1993, focuses on health policy and public health issues. Through the program, journalists specializing in health, or wishing to do so, receive support to do an individually designed project, generally lasting a year. Fellows also meet periodically with each other and with experts in relevant fields. For information on this program and on mini-fellowships, contact the Executive Director, Kaiser Media Fellowships Program, Henry J. Kaiser Family Foundation, 2400 Sand Hill Road, Menlo Park, California 94025, telephone (415) 854-9400.

If you are a physician, you can apply for the Morris Fishbein Fellowship in Medical Editing, sponsored by the American Medical Association. The recipient of this fellowship spends a year working at *JAMA*. Although the fellowship is not in health writing per se, it may appeal to and assist those interested in this realm. Information may be obtained from the *Journal of the American Medical Association,* 515 North State Street, Chicago, Illinois 60610, (312) 464-5000.

Knight Science Journalism Fellowships provide opportunity for journalists covering science, medicine, technology, or the environment to spend nine months at the Massachusetts Institute of Technology. The program is open to freelance writers as well as those employed by the media. Information is available from the Director, Knight Science Journalism Fellowship, Massachusetts Institute of Technology, Room E32-300, 77 Massachusetts Avenue, Cambridge, Massachusetts 02139-4307, telephone (617) 253-3442, fax (617) 258-8100, e-mail mshenry@mit.edu.

The Marine Biological Laboratory Science Writing Fellowships Program, offered each summer at Woods Hole, Massachusetts, provides opportunity to observe and participate in the process of science. Participants normally begin their fellowships with a six-day intensive course introducing research techniques in cell and molecular biology. They can then spend three to seven weeks taking science courses, working in research lab-

15.   Educational Opportunities

oratories, or both. Much of the teaching and research at Woods Hole is biomedically related. Information can be obtained by contacting the Science Writing Fellowships Program, Marine Biological Laboratory, 7 MBL Street, Woods Hole, Massachusetts 02543-1015, telephone (508) 289-7276.

General fellowships for journalists offer a variety of opportunities for health writers. Recipients of Nieman Fellowships for Journalists spend a sabbatical year at Harvard University pursuing courses of study of their own design. During this time, they take and audit courses and participate in a seminar series; they may also work with individual faculty members. Resources available include those at Harvard Medical School and the Harvard School of Public Health. Information may be obtained from the Nieman Foundation, Walter Lippmann House, One Francis Avenue, Cambridge, Massachusetts 02138-2098, telephone (617) 495-2237.

The Alicia Patterson Foundation Fellowship Program for Journalists provides one-year grants to help working journalists pursue independent projects and write articles about them. Since the program was established in 1965, several of the projects have been on health. Applicants must be print journalists with at least five years of professional experience. Information is available from the Alicia Patterson Foundation, 1730 Pennsylvania Avenue, NW, Suite 850, Washington, DC 20006, telephone (202) 393-5995.

The Freedom Forum Media Studies Center offers residential fellowships to media professionals and others. Fellows spend three months to one academic year at the center examining major issues and problems facing mass media and society; commonly, the projects result in books or other major publications. For information, contact the Freedom Forum Media Studies Center, 580 Madison Avenue, New York, New York 10022, telephone (212) 317-6500.

The array of fellowships keeps changing; new fellowships are created, established fellowships evolve, and some are discontinued. Up-to-date listings of many fellowships appear each year in the last issue of the magazine *Editor & Publisher.* Also, more specialized publications, such as the National Association of Science Writers newsletters, *ScienceWriter,* often contain information on fellowships.

Additional Resources

Additional resources for continuing to learn include science writers' briefings, science publications, and journalism magazines.

Especially for health writers who hope to move into broadcasting or wish to strengthen their broadcasting skills, the American Medical Association's Annual Medical Communications and Health Reporting Conference is a resource to consider. Held in the spring, this conference deals largely with television. The conference is more expensive than most held by communications organizations, but scholarships sometimes are available. Information on the conference can be obtained by calling (312) 464-5852 or by writing to the AMA, 515 North State Street, Chicago, Illinois 60610.

Various organizations hold workshops, seminars, or conferences to brief health writers and other journalists on science. For example, each autumn the Council for the Advancement of Science Writing, in collaboration with a university host, holds a several-day New Horizons in Science Briefing. Typically, a considerable proportion of the sessions address biomedical topics. Information is available from the Council for the Advancement of Science Writing, Inc., P.O. Box 404, Greenlawn, New York 11740, telephone (516) 757-5664.

Also, the American Medical Association holds an annual science reporters' conference with presentations on various medical topics. Among the many other groups that present such events or have done so are the American Cancer Society, the American Heart Association, the American Lung Association, and some government agencies concerned with health. Of course, health writers should assess material from these conferences, like that from other sources, for soundness, completeness, and newsworthiness.

Although few health writers have the time and travel funds to attend many such conferences, almost any health writer can draw on other means for keeping up with science, medicine, and related issues. Good written resources in science and medicine include the weekly magazine *Science News,* the news sections of *Science* and *JAMA,* and review and other articles in medical journals. Among less-specialized resources are the major news magazines, which often run well-researched stories on medical topics, and newspapers, some of which publish science or health sections. The broadcast media, through programs such as Nova, can likewise aid in keeping up with medical science. So can World Wide Web sites featuring medical news.

For keeping up on issues and trends in journalism, resources include magazines such as the *American Journalism Review,* the *Columbia Journalism Review,* and the *Quill,* all of which sometimes publish articles on health writing. Health writers working in public information or public relations,

15. Educational Opportunities

especially those in academic settings, may find much of use in *CASE Currents,* published by the Council for Advancement and Support of Education.

And finally, your ongoing search for story ideas and your information-gathering for stories will contribute much to your continuing education. No matter what your initial educational background, and no matter what types of opportunities you pursue to increase your knowledge and skills, health writing is a field in which you will always continue to learn.

REFERENCES

Sources Cited

Adams, Betsy, and John Henkel. 1995. Public affairs specialists: FDA's walking encyclopedias. *FDA Consumer,* May, 23-26.

Albert, Tim. 1995. Press releases need more punch. *Pharmaceutical Marketing,* May, 30-31, 34.

Alternative medicine: Expanding medical horizons. A report to the National Institutes of Health on alternative medical systems and practices in the United States. 1994. Washington, DC: Government Printing Office.

Altman, Lawrence K. 1995. Promises of miracles: News releases go where journals fear to tread. *New York Times,* 10 January, C3.

American Board of Medical Specialties. 1995. *Which medical specialist for you.* Evanston, IL: American Board of Medical Specialties.

American men and women of science. 19th ed. 1994. New Providence, NJ: R.R. Bowker.

American Psychiatric Association. 1994a. *Diagnostic and statistical manual of mental disorders.* 4th ed. Washington, DC: American Psychiatric Association.

American Psychiatric Association. 1994b. *Mental illnesses awareness guide for the media.* Washington, DC: American Psychiatric Association.

American Psychological Association. 1994. *Publication manual of the American Psychological Association.* Washington, DC: American Psychological Association.

Ankrapp, Betty, ed. 1996. *National health directory.* 20th ed. Gaithersburg, MD: Aspen.

Anton, Ted, and Rick McCourt. 1995. *The new science journalists.* New York: Ballantine Books.

Arthritis Foundation. n.d. *The arthritis fact book for the media.* Atlanta: Arthritis Foundation.

Baggot, Teresa. 1992. Personal involvement: Journalists, compassion, and the common good. *Quill,* November/December, 26-7.

Baker, Susan P., Brian O'Neill, Marvin J. Ginsburg, and Guohua Li. 1992. *The injury fact book.* 2d ed. New York: Oxford University Press.

Baldwin, Deborah. 1994. A matter of life and death. *American Journalism Review,* June, 40-5.

References

Banaszynski, Jacqui, and Jean Pieri (photographer). 1987-88. AIDS in the heartland. (Series.) *St. Paul Pioneer Press Dispatch.*

Benenson, Abram S. 1995. *Control of communicable diseases manual.* 16th ed. Washington, DC: American Public Health Association.

Berkow, Robert, ed. 1992. *The Merck manual of diagnosis and therapy.* 16th ed. Rahway, NJ: Merck Research Laboratories.

Bero, Lisa, and Drummond Rennie. 1995. The Cochrane Collaboration: Preparing, maintaining, and disseminating systematic reviews of the effects of health care. *JAMA* 274: 1935-8.

Biagi, Shirley. 1992. *Interviews that work: A practical guide for journalists.* 2d ed. Belmont, CA: Wadsworth.

Biddle, Wayne. 1995. *A field guide to germs.* New York: Henry Holt and Company.

Blum, Deborah, and Mary Knudson, eds. 1997. *A field guide for science writers.* New York: Oxford University Press.

Boisaubin, Eugene V. 1988. Charity, the media, and limited medical resources. *JAMA* 259: 1375-6.

Boyden, Karen, ed. 1994. *Medical and health information directory.* 7th ed. Detroit: Gale Research.

Boyden, Karen, ed. 1996. *Encyclopedia of medical organizations and agencies.* 6th ed. Detroit: Gale Research

Brady, John. 1976. *The craft of interviewing.* New York: Vintage Books.

Breo, Dennis L. 1994. The cancer revolution—from "black box" to "genetic disease." *JAMA* 271: 1452-4.

Brownson, Ann L., ed. 1996. *1996/spring federal staff directory.* Mount Vernon, VA: Staff Directories, Ltd.

Buresh, Bernice, Suzanne Gordon, and Nica Bell. 1991. Who counts in news coverage of health care? *Nursing Outlook* 39: 204-8.

Castelli, Jim. 1990. Welcome to the world of risk communication. *Safety & Health,* August, 68-71.

Christiano, Donna. 1995. Just because it's arthritis . . . *McCall's,* September, E10 ff.

Clayman, Charles B., ed. 1994. *The American Medical Association family medical guide.* 3d ed. New York: Random House.

Cohen, Lynne, and Peter P. Morgan. 1988. Medical dramas and the press: Who benefits from the coverage? *Canadian Medical Association Journal* 139: 657-61.

Cohn, Victor. 1992. Corrective surgery: With science and medical news rapidly expanding, reporters have a responsibility to question facts—and state them with compassion. *Quill,* November/December, 16-8.

Cohn, Victor. 1994. *News and numbers: A guide to reporting statistical claims and controversies in health and other fields.* Rev. ed. Ames: Iowa State University Press.

References

Coleman, Brenda C. (Associated Press.) 1996a. Study: Alzheimer's may be life-long disease. *Bryan-College Station Eagle,* 21 February, A13.

Coleman, Brenda C. (Associated Press.) 1996b. Study finds sex safe for most heart patients. *Bryan-College Station Eagle,* 8 May, A3.

Committee on Risk Perception and Communication. 1989. *Improving risk communication.* Washington, DC: National Academy Press.

Creno, Cathryn. 1992. Sarah's story: Be sure to ask the right questions before writing about the mentally ill. *Quill,* May, 22-25.

Cull, P., ed. 1989. *The sourcebook of medical illustration.* Park Ridge, NJ: Parthenon Publishing Group.

Disabilities Committee of the American Society of Newspaper Editors. 1990. *Reporting on people with disabilities.* (Brochure.) Washington, DC: American Society of Newspaper Editors.

Dorland's illustrated medical dictionary. 28th ed. 1994. Philadelphia: W.B. Saunders.

Dunwoody, Sharon, Elizabeth Crane, and Bonnie Brown, compilers. 1996. *Directory of science communication courses and programs in the United States.* 3d ed. Madison: Center for Environmental Communications and Education Studies, School of Journalism and Mass Communication, University of Wisconsin-Madison.

Eisenberg, David M., Ronald C. Kessler, Cindy Foster, Frances E. Norlock, David R. Calkins, and Thomas L. Delbanco. 1993. Unconventional medicine in the United States: Prevalence, costs, and patterns of use. *New England Journal of Medicine* 328: 246-52.

Elliott, Deni. 1995. Communication, biomedical. I. Media and medicine. In: Reich, Warren Thomas, ed. 1995. *Encyclopedia of bioethics.* Rev. ed. New York: Simon & Schuster Macmillan.

Ferguson, Tom. 1996. *Health online.* Reading, MA: Addison-Wesley.

Fishman, Diane L. 1994. Drug information sources. In: Roper, Fred W., and Jo Anne Boorkman. *Introduction to reference sources in the health sciences.* 3d ed. Metuchen, NJ: Medical Library Association and Scarecrow Press.

Franklin, Jon. 1986. *Writing for story.* New York: New American Library.

Friedman, Sharon M., Sharon Dunwoody, and Carol L. Rogers. 1986. *Scientists and journalists: Reporting science as news.* New York: Free Press.

Fry, Don. 1988. The shocking pictures of Sage: Two newspapers, two answers. *Washington Journalism Review,* April, 35-41.

Gaines, William. 1994. *Investigative reporting for print and broadcast.* Chicago: Nelson-Hall.

Garrett, Laurie. 1989. When death is the end of the story. *Columbia Journalism Review* January/February, 40, 42.

Garrett, Laurie. 1997. Covering infectious diseases. In: Blum, Deborah, and Mary Knudson, eds. *A field guide for science writers.* New York: Oxford University Press.

References

Gastel, Barbara. 1991. A strategy for reviewing books for journals. *BioScience* 41: 635-37.

Gellert, George A., Kathleen V. Higgins, Rosann M. Lowery, and Roberta M. Maxwell. 1994. A national survey of public health officers' interactions with the media. *JAMA* 271: 1285-9.

Gentry, Carol. 1995. The next round of health care hotspots. *Columbia Journalism Review,* July/August, 48.

Gillyatt, Peta. 1996. How to answer your own medical questions. *Harvard Health Letter* (supplement), July, 9-12.

Goldstein, Norm, ed. 1996. *The Associated Press stylebook and libel manual.* 6th trade ed. Reading, MA: Addison-Wesley.

Hamlin, Suzanne. 1995. Health letters scratch out a niche. *New York Times,* 9 August, C1-2.

Haney, Daniel Q. (Associated Press.) 1994. Hospitals battling for family doctors. *Bryan-College Station Eagle,* 29 July, A1, A4.

Harris, Richard F. 1997. Toxics and risk reporting. In: Blum, Deborah, and Mary Knudson, eds. *A field guide for science writers.* New York: Oxford University Press.

Henderson, Randi, and Marjorie Centofanti. 1995. Life as a little person. *Hopkins Medical News,* Spring/Summer, 28-35.

Holm, Kirsten C., ed. 1996. *1997 writer's market.* Cincinnati: Writer's Digest Books.

Houn, Florence, Mary A. Bober, Elmer E. Huerta, Stephen D. Hursting, Stephen Lemon, and Douglas L. Weed. 1995. The association between alcohol and breast cancer: Popular press coverage of research. *American Journal of Public Health* 85: 1082-6.

Huth, Edward J. 1990. *How to write and publish papers in the medical sciences.* 2d ed. Baltimore: Williams & Wilkins.

Imrie, Robert. 1996. Tracking fatal snowmobile accidents. *AP Log,* 28 April, 9.

International Committee of Medical Journal Editors. 1993. Medical journals and the popular media. *New England Journal of Medicine* 328: 1283.

Iverson, Cheryl, Bruce B. Dan, Paula Glitman, Lester S. King, Elizabeth Knoll, Harriet S. Meyer, Kathryn Simmons Raithel, Don Riesenberg, and Roxanne K. Young. 1989. *American Medical Association manual of style.* 8th ed. Baltimore: Williams & Wilkins.

Iverson, Cheryl, Annette Flanagin, Phil Fontanarosa, Richard M. Glass, Paula Glitman, Jane C. Lantz, Harriet S. Meyer, Jeanette M. Smith, Margaret A. Winker, and Roxanne K. Young, 1998. *American Medical Association Manual of Style.* 9th ed. Baltimore: Williams & Wilkins.

Janis, Pam. 1996. In the kitchen: You can't be too clean. *USA Weekend,* January, 5-7, 8.

Jaszczak, Sandra, ed. 1997. *Encyclopedia of associations.* 32d. ed. Detroit: Gale Research.

Kamrin, Michael A., Dolores J. Katz, and Martha L. Walter. 1995. *Reporting on*

References

risk: A journalist's handbook on environmental risk assessment. Los Angeles: Foundation for American Communications.

Kiple, Kenneth F., ed. 1993. *The Cambridge world history of human disease.* New York: Cambridge University Press.

Klass, Perri. 1992. Writing is my best defense. *JAMA* 268: 1191.

Klawans, Harold L. 1991. Hollow victory. *Discover,* December, 80, 82.

Klein, Julie. 1988. The story of Sage. *Quill,* March, 28-34.

Knatterud, Mary E. 1991. Writing with the patient in mind: Don't add insult to injury. *AMWA Journal,* February, 10-7.

Kopelman, Alexander, writer/editor. 1995. *National Writers Union guide to freelance rates and standard practice.* Cincinnati: Writer's Digest Books.

Koren, Gideon, and Naomi Klein. 1991. Bias against negative studies in newspaper reports of medical research. *JAMA* 266: 1824-26.

Kovacs, Beatrice, compiler. 1995. *ALA fingertip guide to national health-information resources.* Chicago: American Library Association.

Krieghbaum, Hillier. 1957. *When doctors meet reporters.* Westport, CT: Greenwood Press.

Lieberman, Trudy. 1993. Focus on health care: A Handbook for journalists. *Columbia Journalism Review,* May/June, 37-44.

Linden, Tom, and Michelle L. Kienholz. 1995. *Dr. Tom Linden's guide to online medicine.* New York: McGraw-Hill.

Maggio, Rosalie. 1991. *The dictionary of bias-free usage: A guide to nondiscriminatory language.* Phoenix: Oryx Press.

Mann, Charles C. 1995. Press coverage: Leaving out the big picture. *Science* 269: 166.

McGraw-Hill encyclopedia of science and technology. 8th ed. 1997. New York: McGraw-Hill.

Medicine and the media: A changing relationship. 1995. Chicago: Robert R. McCormick Tribune Foundation.

Micozzi, Marc S., ed. 1996. *Fundamentals of complementary and alternative medicine.* New York: Churchill Livingstone.

Minick, Phyllis, ed. 1994. *Biomedical communication: Selected AMWA workshops.* Bethesda, MD: American Medical Writers Association.

Mortality Statistics Branch, National Center for Health Statistics. 1996. Mortality patterns—United States, 1993. *Morbidity and Mortality Weekly Report* 45: 161-64.

Morton, Carol Cruzan. 1996. How many ways do science writers love the Internet? *ScienceWriters* (National Association of Science Writers Newsletter), Summer, 21-26.

Moskow, Shirley Blotnick, ed. 1987. *Hunan hand and other ailments: Letters to the New England Journal of Medicine.* Boston: Little, Brown and Company.

National Association of Science Writers. 1996. *Communicating science news: A guide for public information officers, scientists and physicians.* 3d ed. Greenlawn, NY: National Association of Science Writers.

References

National Easter Seal Society. n.d. *Awareness is the first step towards change: Tips for portraying people with disabilities in the media.* (Brochure.) Chicago: National Easter Seal Society.

National Health Information Center. 1997. *Toll-free numbers for health information and Federal health information centers and clearinghouses.* Washington, DC: Office of Disease Prevention and Health Promotion, U.S. Department of Health and Human Services.

National Institute of Neurological Disorders and Stroke. 1994. *Neurological disorders: Voluntary health agencies and other patient resources.* Bethesda, MD: National Institutes of Health.

National Institutes of Health Office of Communications. 1996. *NIH information index.* Bethesda, MD: National Institutes of Health.

National Library of Medicine. 1995. *Guide to NIH HIV/AIDS information services, with selected public health service activities.* Bethesda, MD: National Institutes of Health.

National Library of Medicine. 1996. *Health hotlines: Toll-free numbers from the National Library of Medicine's DIRLINE directory.* Bethesda, MD: National Institutes of Health.

National Safety Council. 1996. *Accident facts.* 1996 ed. Itasca, IL: National Safety Council.

National Stroke Association. 1995. *The stroke/brain attack reporter's handbook.* Englewood, CO: National Stroke Association.

Naythons, Matthew, and Anthony Catsimatides. 1995. *The Internet health, fitness, and medicine yellow pages.* Berkeley, CA: Osborne McGraw-Hill.

Neergaard, Lauran. (Associated Press.) 1995. A pox on a common childhood disease: FDA approves the first vaccine for chickenpox. *Bryan-College Station Eagle,* 18 March, A6.

The official ABMS directory of board certified medical specialists. 29th ed. 1997. New Providence, NJ: Marquis Who's Who.

Oleckno, William A. 1995. Guidelines for improving risk communication in environmental health. *Journal of Environmental Health* 58: 20-3.

Oxman, Andrew D., Gordon H. Guyatt, Deborah J. Cook, Roman Jaeschke, Nancy Heddle, and Jana Keller. 1993. An index of scientific quality for health reports in the lay press. *Journal of Clinical Epidemiology* 46: 987-1001.

Paul, Nora. 1995. *Computer assisted research: A guide to tapping online information.* St. Petersburg, FL: Poynter Institute for Media Studies. (Available online at http://www.nando.net/prof/poynter/chome.html)

Paulos, John Allen. 1995. *A mathematician reads the newspaper.* New York: Basic-Books.

Phillips, David P., Elliot J. Kanter, Bridget Bednarczyk, and Patricia L. Tastad. 1991. Importance of the lay press in the transmission of medical knowledge to the scientific community. *New England Journal of Medicine* 325: 1180-3.

References

PhRMA. 1996. *Reporter's handbook for the prescription drug industry.* Washington, DC: Pharmaceutical Research and Manufacturers of America.

Physicians' desk reference. 51st ed. 1997. Montvale, NJ: Medical Economics Company.

Reddick, Randy, and Elliot King. 1997. *The online journalist: Using the Internet for research and reporting.* 2d ed. Fort Worth, TX: Harcourt Brace College Publishers.

Reich, Warren Thomas, ed. 1995. *Encyclopedia of bioethics.* Rev. ed. New York: Simon & Schuster Macmillan.

Research and Training Center on Independent Living. 1993. *Guidelines for reporting and writing about people with disabilities.* 4th ed. (Brochure.) Lawrence, KS: Research and Training Center on Independent Living.

Rodgers, Joann Ellison, and William C. Adams. 1994. *Media guide for academics.* Los Angeles: Foundation for American Communications.

Roper, Fred W., and Jo Anne Boorkman, compiler. 1994. *Introduction to reference sources in the health sciences.* 3d ed. Metuchen, NJ: Medical Library Association and Scarecrow Press.

Roueché, Berton. 1982. *The medical detectives.* New York: Washington Square Press.

Roueché, Berton. 1986. *The medical detectives, volume II.* New York: Washington Square Press.

Roueché, Berton. 1995. *The man who grew two breasts and other tales of medical detection.* New York: Truman Talley Books/Plume.

Rowan, Katherine E. 1990. Strategies for explaining complex science news. *Journalism Educator* 45(2): 25-31.

Rubin, Rita, and Harrison L. Rogers, Jr. 1994. *Under the microscope: The relationship between physicians and the news media.* Nashville: The Freedom Forum First Amendment Center at Vanderbilt University.

Sachs, Jessica Snyder. 1996. A fix for migraines. *Health,* January/February, 86-8.

Sapolsky, Robert M. 1990. Why you feel crummy when you're sick. *Discover,* July, 66-70.

Schwartz, Marilyn, and the Task Force on Bias-Free Usage of the Association of American University Presses. 1995. *Guidelines for bias-free writing.* Bloomington: Indiana University Press.

Schwitzer, Gary J. 1992. Doctoring the news: Miracle cures, video press releases, and TV medical reporting. *Quill,* November/December, 19-21.

Scully, Celia G., and Thomas J. Scully. 1986. *How to make money writing about fitness and health.* Cincinnati: Writer's Digest Books.

Shaw, Donald L., and Paul Van Nevel. 1967. The informative value of medical science news. *Journalism Quarterly* 44: 548.

Shepard, Alicia C. 1996. Show and print. *American Journalism Review,* March, 40-44.

Smith, Martin J. 1993. Media as God: Many stories generate compassion, but good ones spread it around. *Quill,* November/December, 22-23.

References

Society for Neuroscience. 1993. *Brain facts: A primer on the brain and nervous system.* Washington, DC: Society for Neuroscience.

Stedman's medical dictionary. 26th ed. 1995. Baltimore: Williams & Wilkins.

Steele, Bob. 1992. Doing ethics: How a Minneapolis journalist turned a difficult situation into a human triumph. *Quill,* November/December, 28-30.

Stempel, Guido H. III, and Hugh M. Culbertson. 1984. The prominence and dominance of news sources in newspaper medical coverage. *Journalism Quarterly* 61: 671-76.

Stephenson, Joan. 1995. Medical technology watchdog plays unique role in quality assessment. *JAMA* 274: 999-1001.

Stephenson, Joan. 1996. "Mini-med schools" offer lay public lessons in the science of medicine. *JAMA* 275: 897-9.

Stone, John. 1992. Night wanderings. *New York Times Magazine,* 19 January, 14, 16.

Strunk, William Jr., and E.B. White. 1979. *The elements of style.* 3d ed. New York: Macmillan.

Taubes, Gary. 1996a. Science journals go wired. *Science* 271: 764-66.

Taubes, Gary. 1996b. Looking for the evidence in medicine. *Science* 272: 22-24.

Thomas, Lewis. 1974. Germs. In: *The lives of a cell: Notes of a biology watcher.* New York: Viking Press.

Thomas, Patricia. 1993. The best medical reference books. *Harvard Health Letter* (supplement), November, 9-12.

Trafford, Abigail. 1997. Critical coverage of public health and government. In: Blum, Deborah, and Mary Knudson, eds. *A field guide for science writers.* New York: Oxford University Press.

Travis, J. 1995. New drug staves off osteoporosis. *Science News,* 24 June, 388.

Travis, J. 1996. Second protein opens cells to HIV's entry. *Science News,* 11 May, 293.

Ullmann, John, and Jan Colbert, eds. 1991. *The reporter's handbook: An investigator's guide to documents and techniques.* 2d ed. New York: St. Martin's Press.

Utts, Jessica M. 1996. *Seeing through statistics.* Belmont, CA: Wadsworth.

Verghese, Abraham. 1994. *My own country: A doctor's story.* New York: Simon & Schuster.

Waldron, Brian J. 1993. Tyranny and cruelty. *Discover,* August, 90-2.

Walsh-Childers, Kim. 1994a. Newspaper influence on health policy development. *Newspaper Research Journal* 15(3): 89-104.

Walsh-Childers, Kim. 1994b. "A death in the family"—a case study of newspaper influence on health policy development. *Journalism Quarterly* 71: 820-9.

Ward, Darrell E. 1995. *The cancer handbook: A guide for the nonspecialist.* Columbus: Ohio State University Press.

Weaver, Daniel C. 1994. The secret in the marrow. *Discover,* January, 26, 28-9.

Weinberg, Steve. 1996. *The reporter's handbook: An investigator's guide to docu-*

ments and techniques. 3d ed. New York: St Martin's Press.

West, Bernadette, Peter M. Sandman, and Michael R. Greenberg. 1995. *The reporter's environmental handbook.* New Brunswick, NJ: Rutgers University Press.

What you need to know about cancer. 1996. *Scientific American* (special issue), September.

Wilkes, Michael S., and Richard L. Kravitz. 1992. Medical researchers and the media: Attitudes toward public dissemination of research. *JAMA* 268: 999-1003.

Williams, Mark E. 1995. *The American Geriatrics Society's complete guide to aging and health.* New York: Harmony Books.

Witte, Florence M., and Nancy Dew Taylor, eds. 1997. *Essays for biomedical communicators: Part 2 of selected AMWA workshops.* Bethesda, MD: American Medical Writers Association.

Zinsser, William. 1994. *On writing well: An informal guide to writing nonfiction.* 5th ed. New York: HarperCollins.

Sources of Additional Help or Perspective

AAAS launches on-line service for research news. 1996. *Science* 272: 1366.

Adams, R.M. 1993. Rx for health writing. *The Writer,* June, 22-3.

Albert, Tim. 1993. How to do it: Set up a newsletter. *British Medical Journal* 305: 631-5.

Albert, Tim, with Joy Noel Tavalino. 1995. *Medical journalism: The writer's guide to getting published.* New York: Radcliffe Medical Press.

Albrecht, Laura J. 1992. A dose of information: What are your patients reading? *Texas Medicine,* September, 36-42.

Altman, Lawrence K. 1993. Bringing the news to the public: The role of the media. *Annals of the New York Academy of Sciences* 703: 200-9.

American College of Obstetricians and Gynecologists. 1996. *Issues in women's health media kit.* Washington, DC: American College of Obstetricians and Gynecologists.

American Veterinary Medical Association. 1996. *1996 media guide to veterinary sources and information.* Schaumberg, IL: American Veterinary Medical Association.

Angell, Marcia, and Jerome P. Kassirer. 1991. The Ingelfinger Rule revisited. *New England Journal of Medicine* 325: 1371-3.

Angell, Marcia, and Jerome P. Kassirer. 1994. Clinical research—what should the public believe? *New England Journal of Medicine* 331: 189-90.

Atkin, Charles, and Lawrence Wallack, eds. 1990. *Mass communication and public health: Complexities and conflicts.* Newbury Park, CA: Sage Publications.

Aumente, Jerome. 1995. A medical breakthrough: Once the province of correspondents without a clue, network medical reporting now showcases

References

specialists who use their expertise to sort through the confusing welter of reports, studies, developments and "cures." *American Journalism Review,* December, 26-33.

Blakeslee, Alton. 1994. Late night thoughts about science writing. *Quill,* November/December, 35-8.

Bonner, Staci. 1995. Hard facts on fact checking. *Writer's Digest,* August, 37-9.

Breo, Dennis L. 1989. Meet Vic Cohn—dean of American science writers. *JAMA* 262: 968-70.

Brown, Martin L., and Arnold L. Potosky. 1990. The presidential effect: The public health response to media coverage about Ronald Reagan's colon cancer episode. *Public Opinion Quarterly* 54: 317-29.

Burkett, Warren. 1986. *News reporting: Science, medicine, and high technology.* Ames: Iowa State University Press.

Caplan, Arthur L. 1989. The concepts of health and disease. In: Veatch, Robert M., ed. *Medical ethics.* Boston: Jones and Bartlett.

Caudill, Edward, and Paul Ashdown. 1989. The New England Journal of Medicine as news source. *Journalism Quarterly* 66: 458-62.

Centers for Disease Control and Prevention. 1994. Programs for the prevention of suicide among adolescents and young adults; Suicide contagion and the reporting of suicide: Recommendations from a national workshop. *Morbidity and Mortality Weekly Report* 43 (No. RR-6): 1-18.

Creno, Cathryn. 1992. How do you say it? Advice for covering the disabilities beat. *Quill,* May, 19-20.

Dahir, Mubarak S. 1995. Writing science and medical nonfiction: It's easier than you think. *Writer's Digest,* November, 29-31.

Day, Robert A. 1994. *How to write and publish a scientific paper.* 4th ed. Phoenix: Oryx Press.

Ensminger, Audrey H., M.E. Ensminger, James E. Konlande, and John R.K. Robson. 1994. *Foods and nutrition encyclopedia.* 2d ed. Boca Raton, FL: CRC Press.

Entwistle, Vikki. 1995. Reporting research in medical journals and newspapers. *British Medical Journal* 310: 920-3.

Ferguson, John H. 1996. On-line medicine @nih.gov. *JAMA* 275: 94.

Fischer, Heinz-Dietrich. 1992. *Medicine, media and morality: Pulitzer Prize-winning writings on health-related topics.* Malabar, FL: Krieger Publishing Company.

Garner, Jean. 1993. A window on health. [Newsletters as sources.] *Columbia Journalism Review,* July/August, 14-5.

Gastel, Barbara. 1983. *Presenting science to the public.* Philadelphia: ISI Press.

Gersh, Debra. 1993. Writing about your own ordeal. *Editor & Publisher,* 20 February, 12-3, 42.

Glanz, Karen, and Haiou Yang. 1996. Communicating about risk of infectious diseases. *JAMA* 275: 253-6.

Goldsmith, Marsha F. 1995. Directed to defend its raison d'etre, NIH holds communications conference. *JAMA* 273: 761, 763-64.

Harby, Karla. 1993. Doctors as reporters: A check-up. *Columbia Journalism Review,* July/August, 11-13.

Health Care Financing Administration. 1995. *1995 HCFA Statistics.* Washington, DC: Government Printing Office.

Husten, Larry. 1994. Understanding risk: Tricky business. *Harvard Health Letter* (supplement), October, 9-12.

Jamieson, Kathleen Hall. 1995. Health messages: News media might have side effects. *ScienceWriters,* Spring, 1-4.

Jimenez, Sherry L.M. 1991. Consumer journalism: A unique nursing opportunity. *Image: Journal of Nursing Scholarship* 23(1): 47-9.

Kaiser Family Foundation. 1996. Covering the epidemic: AIDS in the news media, 1985-1996. *Columbia Journalism Review* (supplement), July/August.

Kassirer, Jerome P., and Marcia Angell. 1994. Violations of the embargo and a new policy on early publicity. *New England Journal of Medicine* 330: 1608-09.

Kessler, Lauren. 1989. Women's magazines' coverage of smoking related health hazards. *Journalism Quarterly* 66: 316-22, 445.

Kinsella, James. 1989. *Covering the plague: AIDS and the American media.* New Brunswick, NJ: Rutgers University Press.

Kirkwood, William G., and Dan Brown. 1995. Public communication about the causes of disease: The rhetoric of responsibility. *Journal of Communication* 45(1): 55-76.

Klaidman, Stephen. 1991. *Health in the headlines: The stories behind the stories.* New York: Oxford University Press.

Krossel, Martin. 1988. "Handicapped heroes" and the knee-jerk press. *Columbia Journalism Review,* May/June, 46-47.

Lane, Dorothy S., Anthony P. Polednak, and Mary Ann Burg. 1989. The impact of media coverage of Nancy Reagan's experience of breast cancer screening. *American Journal of Public Health* 79: 1551-52.

Lang, Thomas A. 1994. Developing patient education handouts. In: Minick, Phyllis, ed. *Biomedical communication: Selected AMWA workshops.* Bethesda, MD: American Medical Writers Association.

Lathrop, Douglas. 1995. Challenging perceptions: Disability press sets example: Eschews pity, hero worship for images of people leading independent, active lives. *Quill,* July/August, 36-38.

Lewton, Kathleen Larey. 1995. *Public relations in health care: A guide for professionals.* 2d ed. Chicago: American Hospital Publishing.

Lippert, Joan. 1992. Writing a publishable health article. *The Writer,* March, 17-20.

Maibach, Edward, and Roxanne Louiselle Parrott, eds. 1995. *Designing health messages: Approaches from communication theory and public health practice.* Thousand Oaks, CA: Sage Publications.

Mahaney, Francis X. Jr. 1992. Television's news doctors: How they operate.

References

Journal of the National Cancer Institute 84: 569-70.

Medical news: How to assess the latest breakthrough. 1997. *Consumer Reports,* June, 62-63.

Medicine and the media. (Multi-authored series.) 1996. *Lancet* 347: 1087-90, 1163-66, 1240-43, 1308-11, 1382-86, 1459-63, 1533-55, 1600-03.

Moore, Mike, ed. 1989. *Health risks and the press: Perspectives on media coverage of risk assessment and health.* Washington, DC: The Media Institute.

National Depressive and Manic-Depressive Association. 1996. *Advancing Mental Health: A Guide for Journalists.* Chicago: NDMDA.

National Institute on Deafness and Other Communication Disorders Information Clearinghouse. *Directory 1994—Resources for deafness and other communication disorders.* Washington, DC: NIDCD Information Clearinghouse.

Nelkin, Dorothy. 1985. Managing biomedical news. *Social Research* 52: 625-46.

Nelson, Jack A., ed. 1994. *The disabled, the media, and the information age.* Westport, CT: Greenwood Press.

Nowak, Rachel. 1995. Publicity fears cancel gene talk. *Science* 270: 909-10.

Office of Disease Prevention and Health Promotion. 1991. *Mass media and health: Opportunities for improving the nation's health.* Washington, DC: U.S. Department of Health and Human Services.

Otten, Alan L. 1992. The influence of the mass media on health policy. *Health Affairs* 11(4): 111-18.

Paul Raeburn offers a wire-service view of science writing. 1994. *ScienceWriters,* Fall, 9-12.

Perl, Rebecca. 1995. Covering tobacco: A handbook for journalists. *Columbia Journalism Review,* March/April, 33-40.

Relman, Arnold S. 1981. The Ingelfinger Rule. *New England Journal of Medicine* 305: 824-26.

Rich, Carole. 1989. Don't call them "spry." *Quill,* February, 12-13, 38.

Rourk, Malcolm H. Jr., Robert A. Hock, Joye S. Pursell, David Jones, and Alexander Spock. 1981. The news media and the doctor-patient relationship. *New England Journal of Medicine* 305: 1278-80.

Roush, Wade. 1995. "Fat hormone" poses hefty problem for journal embargo. *Science* 269: 627.

Schear, Stuart. 1994. Covering health care: Politics or people? *Columbia Journalism Review,* May/June, 36-37.

Schenker, Jonathan. 1991. Use of patients as health care sources. *Public Relations Journal,* July, 23-25.

Schwager, Edith. 1991. *Medical English usage and abusage.* Phoenix: Oryx Press.

Schwitzer, Gary. 1992. The magical medical media tour. *JAMA* 267: 1969-71.

Sibbison, Jim. 1985. Pushing new drugs—can the press kick the habit? *Columbia Journalism Review,* July/August, 52-54.

Sibbison, Jim. 1988. Covering medical "breakthroughs." *Columbia Journalism Review,* July/August, 36-39.

References

Sikorski, Robert, and Richard Peters. 1997. Oncology ASAP: Where to find reliable cancer information on the Internet. *JAMA* 277: 1431-32.

Smith, Tori. 1992. "Dr. Dan" Haney: the AP's GP. *AP World,* March/April, 9-10.

Sontag, Susan. 1978. *Illness as metaphor.* New York: Farrar, Straus and Giroux.

Sontag, Susan. 1989. *AIDS and its metaphors.* New York: Farrar, Straus and Giroux.

Stephenson, Joan. 1995. Journal's aversion to prepublication publicity silences researchers at human genetics meeting. *JAMA* 274: 1666.

Stolberg, Sheryl. 1993. Confessions of a first-year medical writer. *Nieman Reports,* Winter, 6-7 ff.

Stothers, William. 1992. Disabilities, the disabled, and the media. *Quill,* May, 16-19.

Wahl, Otto F. 1995. *Media madness: Public images of mental illness.* New Brunswick, NJ: Rutgers University Press.

Warner, Kenneth E., Linda M. Goldenhar, and Catherine G. McLaughlin. 1992. Cigarette advertising and magazine coverage of the hazards of smoking: A statistical analysis. *New England Journal of Medicine* 326: 305-09.

Ziporyn, Terra. 1988. *Disease in the popular American press: The case of diphtheria, typhoid fever, and syphilis, 1870-1920.* New York: Greenwood Press.

INDEX

Index

Brand names, 125–26
Breakthroughs, 123
Business Press Educational Foundation,
    199

C

*Cambridge World History of Human
    Disease,* 13
Canadian Medical Association Journal, 14
Cancer, information sources on, 138–39,
    199
Career options. *See also* Genres
    in freelance writing, 182–84
    in health writing, 184–85
    in print, broadcast, and electronic
        media, 177–80
    in public information and public re-
        lations, 180–81
Case, patient versus, 123
CASE Currents, 203
Causality, 79
Centers for Disease Control and Preven-
    tion (CDC), 17, 37–38, 128, 140,
    150, 155
Chronicle of Higher Education, 184
Clinician's Research Digest, 17
Clusters, 78
Cochrane Collaboration, 146
Codes of ethics, 160–64
Columbia Journalism Review, 148, 202
Compare to/compare with, 130
Comprise, 130
Computerized information sources,
    9–10, 26–27. *See also* Online re-
    sources
Conclusions, 92–93
Conferences, 44–46, 202–3
Confidence intervals, 77
Confidentiality, 168
Conflicts of interest, 166–67
Consistency, 69
Context, 100–101, 104, 106, 109, 110. *See
    also* Big picture evaluation
Continual/continuous, 130
Controlled clinical trial, 70
Correlation, 79
Cost evaluation, 81
Council for Advancement and Support
    of Education, 203
Council for the Advancement of Science
    Writing (CASW), 198, 202

Council of Biology Editors Inc. (CBE),
    190–91
Courses. *See* Educational Opportunities
Criterion/criteria, 130
Cross-sectional studies, 71
Current Contents, 17

D

Degrees, 123–24
Deja News, 63
Depth reporting, 102, 105, 111–13
DIALOG, 40
Die of, 124
Different from, 131
DIRLINE, 29–30, 40
Disabilities, writing about, 119–21
Diseases
    capitalization of names of, 123
    information sources on, 137–44
    writing about, 119–21
Dorland's Illustrated Medical Dictionary, 11
Double-blind clinical trial, 70
Dr. Tom Linden's Guide to Online Medicine,
    59
Drugs, generic and brand names of,
    125–26

E

ECRI, 145–46
Editor & Publisher, 184
Educational institutions as information
    sources, 10, 42–43
Educational opportunities
    courses and programs, 195–98
    fellowships, 199–201
    internships, 198–99
Effect/affect, 129–30
E-mail. *See also* Online resources
    for accessing institutional informa-
        tion sources, 33–34
    cautions regarding, 63
    for checking accuracy, 95
    for conducting interviews, 49, 62
    interviewing via, 50, 53
Embargoes on journal articles, 22–26
Employers, 165–66
Encyclopedia of Associations, 32, 40
Encyclopedia of Bioethics, 13, 160
Endings, 92–93
Environmental Protection Agency (EPA),
    155

Index

Index

Index

News releases, 99–102, 108–11
News stories, 99–102, 103–7
NEXIS, 40
Nieman Fellowships for Journalists, 201
Nobel Prize, 132
Numbers
  averages, 75
  clusters, 78
  evaluating and presenting, 73–78, 92
  health-related rates, 73–74
  percent change, 75–76
  relative risk, 76
  response rates, 74–75
  statistical power, 77–78
  statistical significance, 76–77
  using statisticians, 73

O
Obituaries, 118
Occupational Safety and Health Administration (OSHA), 155
Office of Alternative Medicine (OAM), 147
Office of Disease Prevention and Health Promotion (ODPHP), 39
Office of Medical Applications for Research (OMAR), 145
Official ABMS Directory of Board Certified Medical Specialists, 54
Online resources. *See also* Computerized information sources; E-mail; World Wide Web sites/addresses
  discussion groups, 63
  institutional, 33–34
  Internet guidebooks, 59–60
  medical conference information, 44
  medical periodical, 17
  researcher home pages, 51
Ophthalmologist, 128
Optician, 128
Optometrist, 128
Orientation, 90
Overview articles, 114, 115–16

P
Patient, versus case, 123
Patient interviews, 55–57
Peer review, 21–22
Percent changes, 75–76
Periodicals. *See* Medical periodicals
Personal-experience articles, 117

Pharmaceutical companies as information source, 43–44
Pharmaceutical Research and Manufacturers of America (PhRMA), 44, 146
Phenomenon/phenomena, 130
Photographs, 91. *See also* Illustrations
Physician, 127
Physicians' Desk Reference, 12
Points of entry, 90
Pre-publication publicity, 22–26
Prevalence, 126–27
Prevalence rates, 74, 126–27
Privacy, 168
Probability values, 77
Professional organizations, 187–93. *See also specific organization*
Profiles, 117
ProfNet, 48, 51, 184
Programs. *See* Educational Opportunities
Prospective research, 70–71
Psychiatrist, 128
Psychologist, 128
Publication sites, 165–66
Public information writing, 180–81
Public Relations Society of America (PRSA), 191-92
Public relations writing, 3, 181–82
P values, 77

Q
Quill, 160, 202
Quotations, 91–92

R
Randomized clinical trial, 70
Readers' Guide to Periodical Literature, 9
Reference books. *See* Information sources
Reflected light, 117
Relative risk, 76
Reporter's Environmental Handbook, The, 156
Reporter's Handbook: An Investigator's Guide to Documents and Techniques, 111, 112
Reporter's Handbook for the Prescription Drug Industry, 44
Reporting on Risk: A Journalist's Handbook on Environmental Risk Assessment, 156
Research and Training Center on Inde-

Index

Index